Breathe
for Life

I dedicate this book to my very special teacher, Chris Stansfield,
who was the first person to teach me to breathe deeply.

I'd also like to dedicate this book to my other teachers whose passion
and dedication to breathing have inspired me for life:

Rosemarie Holmes—for teaching me that "Breath is Life."

Valda Moore—for showing me different dimensions of breathing.

Chin Moi Chow—for educating me about the technical side of breathing,
and for all her help with this book.

To each and every person I have taught, you are all a part of this book
because you were also teaching me more about breathing
through your questions, insights and realizations.

Breathe for Life

How to Reduce Stress & Enhance Your Fitness

Sophie Gabriel

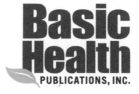

Basic Health
PUBLICATIONS, INC.

The information contained in this book is based upon the research and personal and professional experiences of the author. It is not intended as a substitute for consulting with your physician or other health care provider. Any attempt to diagnose and treat an illness should be done under the direction of a health care professional.

The publisher does not advocate the use of any particular health care protocol but believes the information in this book should be available to the public. The publisher and author are not responsible for any adverse effects or consequences resulting from the use of the suggestions, preparations, or procedures discussed in this book. Should the reader have any questions concerning the appropriateness of any procedures or preparation mentioned, the author and the publisher strongly suggest consulting a professional health care advisor.

Published by
Basic Health Publications, Inc.
8200 Boulevard East
North Bergen, NJ 07047
1-201-868-8336

Published by arrangement with Hardie Grant Books, South Yarra, Australia.

Library of Congress Cataloging-in-Publication Data

Gabriel, Sophie, 1962–
    Breathe for life / Sophie Gabriel.
        p. ; cm.
Includes index.
    ISBN 1-59120-002-4
1. Respiration. 2. Breathing exercises.
    [DNLM: 1. Breathing Exercises. 2. Health Promotion.
3. Teaching—methods. WB 541 G118b 2002] I. Title.
    RA782.G15 2002
    613'.192—dc21

                                    2002000907

Typesetting: Gary A. Rosenberg
Cover Design: The Great American Art Company

Printed in the United States of America

10   9   8   7   6   5   4   3   2   1

Contents

Contributors

Contributing writers

I would like to say a special thank you to the following people for their contributions to the manuscript:

Dr. Chin Moi Chow had a huge input into the whole manuscript from the beginning until the end. Erica Scott assisted with the manuscript and wrote the 10-step instructions for massage. Angela Carroll and Emma, Annie, Linda, Glen, Loanna, Tony and Sue contributed to the section on labor, as did midwife Chris Ferlazzo. My sister, Marie, helped me in the early stages, and her statements are included in the introduction. Joan Lewis proofread my manuscript and provided a quote and Ann Hewitt also helped with the manuscript.

Scientific and medical contributors

The following medical experts proofread relevant parts of the manuscript:

Dr. Chin Moi Chow M.Sc., Ph.D.

Dr. Chin Moi Chow is a senior lecturer in the School of Exercise and Sports Science at the University of Sydney. Her Ph.D. and post-doctoral research focused on breathing mechanisms related to breathing cessation in sudden infant death syndrome and breathing cessation during sleep respectively. Dr. Chow devoted much of her earlier teaching career to respiratory physiology and more recently to exercise physiology. Currently, she is conducting research in breathing, sleep and sports performance.

Ellen Dickson B.Sc. (Applied Biology, CNAA)

Ellen Dickson's experience includes teaching anatomy and physiology, as well as organizing Flexible Delivery Anatomy and Physiology Training Packages for RMIT. She was also Acting Head of the Department of Health and Clinical Sciences, RMIT.

Dr. Nicos Kokotsis FACE, MBBS, B.Med.Sc.

Dr. Kokotsis is a staff specialist at the Austin Hospital in the Department. of Emergency Medicine. He is also a consultant for both the international Medical Retrieval and the Intensive Care Unit at Maroondah Hospital.

Damon Kendrick B.Sc.(med)(hons) Sport Science, Grad Dip Ed & T, Grad Dip Sport Mmt

Damon Kendrick trained as a sport scientist and practiced as an exercise physiologist for many years, performing fitness assessments on over 30,000 individuals. He is now Academic Coordinator of the Melbourne College of Natural Medicine where he also teaches anatomy, physiology, biochemistry and sports injury management.

I would like to acknowledge that all the medical proofreaders have had a significant influence on the technical aspect of this book, and they were all involved in writing parts of the following sections:

- What is a good/bad quality breath? What happens when I breathe shallowly? The benefits of breathing deeply?
- The causes of faulty and shallow breathing
- Training the breath
- Healthy natural breathing and signs of respiratory distress
- Breathing in and out of the nose
- Breathing patterns
- Flexibility and stretching

- Massage
- Breathing programs
- Breathing training for singers and musicians
- Breathing for sports and movement
- Coping with pain
- Breathing during labor
- Insomnia
- Asthma

All medical and scientific contributors had input into the body and the breath, but it was written mainly by Dr. Chow, including the technical definitions of breathing—inhalation/exhalation, shallow breathing and abdominal/diaphragmatic breathing. Every effort has been made to ensure that all the information in this book is correct; however, I bear full responsibility for any factual errors that may appear in this work.

Contributing books

The following books have impressed me, and certain quotes or information from some of them have been included in this book.

Bragg, Patricia and Paul, *Super Power Breathing,* Health Science, USA

Dillner, Luisa and Tom Snow, *The Human Body,* Wishing Well Books, Victoria, 1997

Hendler, Sheldon, *The Oxygen Breakthrough,* Simon and Schuster Inc., New York, USA, 1990

Hendricks, Gay, *Conscious Breathing,* Bantam Books, USA, 1995

Le Boyer, Frederick, *Birth Without Violence,* Wild Woodhouse Ltd, Great Britain, 1995

Speads, Carola, *Ways to Better Breathing,* Felix Morrow, New York, 1986

Acknowledgments

Over the last 10 years, there have been so many people who have supported and encouraged me and I would like to thank:

Evros and Meropi Gabrielson, Marie Gabrielson, Peter and George, Poppy, Steven, John and Georgie Gabrielson, Ronald Bradley, Di McCloud, Brian Looker, Christine Amor, Carol Van Miltenburg, Brook Ramage, Maz O'Connor, Linda Kedzlie, Sophie Norton Smith, Maddison Hackett, Ken Roche, Richard and Bonnie Diaz, Bob Thomas and Bob Delmonteque, Patricia Bragg (and the late Paul Bragg), Aslan Avdi, Suzy Daley, Jacques and Rhonda Khoury, Margaret Hill, Barbara Key, Kevin Jacobsen, Jamie Turner, Mary and John Bruniges, Peter Edwards, Maureen Williams, Haizel Bartlett, Jill O'Connor, Carolyn McDougall, Dr. Peter, Dr. Ahmed and Genivieve, Dr. Beales, Marion and Nick, Kelly O'Neil, Anthony Edwards and Ransley Mascurine.

To my publisher, Sandy Grant, thank you for your vision for my book. A huge thank you must also go to Tracy O'Shaughnessy, Heather Millar, Kirsty Manning, Julie Pinkham and Catherine Aldred. I would also like to express my appreciation and gratitude to my agents, Jacinta Di Mase and Jenny Darling.

Foreword

The Lord God formed the man from the dust of ground and breathed into his nostrils the breath of life, and the man became a living being.

Genesis 2:7

This book captures Sophie's philosophy to live a life that is healthy and hearty—to breathe is to nourish and sustain life. She has practiced her philosophies from a very young age and her teaching methods for Breathing Training prompted the conception of *Breathe for Life*.

Sophie justly has her focus on breathing. We utter our first cries as newborns, taking in that first deep breath to inflate our previously liquid-filled lungs. From then on, breathing must continue every minute of our lives, awake or asleep.

Breathing is an unconscious act. We breathe on demand, by a need signaled from within the body. Breathing is to satisfy the oxygen needs of the majority of millions of living cells in our bodies. We naturally breathe more when we are physically active. The drive to breathe lies with the need to supply oxygen to the working muscles and the need to remove carbon dioxide from our bodies. The drive is dictated by our bodily needs.

Behavior has a strong control over breathing. Even a child knows instinctively to play on the mother's emotions by an exhaustive cry that is associated with "exhaustive" breathing—hyperventilation. Our emotions can turn our normal relaxed breathing into an unconscious heightened state of breathing that may become a life-long trait. The impact of hyperventilation is huge. It can lead to agitation, irritability, the sensation of pins and needles and fatigue. Behavioral modification of breathing does not need to cause systematic or psychological harm. Our speech and the control of our voices simply reflect the way we control our breathing. And this control is so powerful as to produce the greatest sensation—as found in singing. Breathing is a trainable act.

There are many individuals who are unaware of their abnormal breathing pattern and behavior. Such breathing habits may have been acquired on an occasion that saw trauma, tragedy, loss of a loved one or situations of emotional disturbance. These unhealthy breathing habits can be broken and reversed.

Sophie's breathing techniques are physiologically sound. *Breathe for Life* lets you get in touch with your breathing, your respiratory muscles and rib cage. The teaching guide comes with a preamble of her experience, followed with step-by-step instructions.

Breathe for Life offers you the essence of calmness, relaxation and the feeling of being in control. You will enjoy it.

Chin Moi Chow, Ph.D.
Respiratory Physiologist
University of Sydney

An important note to all readers

The information in this book is intended for everyone who wants to learn techniques to improve their breathing. The motivation for wanting to improve breathing methods can be a variety of factors, including a specific purpose.

It is crucial from the outset to state that disease can create changes in breathing. Therefore, people with diseases such as asthma, emphysema and heart disease must discuss any form of training with their doctors or specialists. Also, those who have a disease should assume that their shortness of breath and worsening of their problem are always due to worsening of their disease. They should seek medical attention immediately and not commence breathing exercises in the hope that they improve. (People have died in these circumstances.)

You may feel you are basically healthy, but discover at some stage that your breathing is obviously rapid, and that you are breathing more than 16 times a minute. At this point, *do not* proceed with the breathing exercises outlined in this or any other book. *It is crucial that you consult your doctor to exclude an organic disease.* Feeling breathless without physical exertion doesn't always mean that you are unfit, but is often an early sign of disease.

I strongly advise everybody to check with their doctors before embarking on the advice given in this book—especially pregnant women, or anyone requiring medical attention.

Breath is life

Breathing right is unquestionably the single most important thing you can do to improve your life. It will help you to live a longer, more energetic and stress-free life.

Dr. Sheldon Hendler, *The Oxygen Breakthrough*

Breath is life. . .it literally is. It is the beginning of life, it sustains life, and when it is gone, no life remains. Yet so many of us take it for granted. It's only when something goes wrong with our breathing, or if we require specialized breathing training for sports, singing, or a medical condition, that we stop to even *think* about the way we breathe.

Wouldn't you want to find the time to stop and think about the way you breathe if I were to tell you that by improving the quality of their breathing, some people have been rewarded with:

- better sleeping patterns
- a sense of well-being and calm
- an enhanced ability to handle stress
- the ability to relax at will

I am constantly asked how I became involved in breathing training, and so I'd like to share with you how I discovered the world of the breath and just how important good quality breathing training is. . . .

When I was 14 years old, I began to study karate with Chris Stansfield, a special person and instructor who viewed martial arts holistically—that is, he used it to teach character development as much as self-defense. He taught his students self-respect and discipline as well as correct technique—and he also taught me how to breathe deeply.

From the moment I was introduced to the art of breathing, I was fascinated. It felt like such freedom to *consciously* move that gentle yet powerful life force through my body. Now, 20 years later, if I focus and take a long, slow, deep breath, I can still experience the same exhilarating sensation I felt back then.

As a teenage girl studying karate, I was surrounded by men who somehow seemed oblivious to pain. I had to learn how to handle the pain, or drop out. I loved the world of martial arts, and Chris Stansfield was just the person to teach me all I needed to know. His teachings about mental discipline and breathing techniques helped me to withstand the pain and survive in the world of martial arts. By the time I was 15, I had already started developing my breathing for exercise and began applying different breathing techniques to help overcome pain and increase my stamina and fitness level.

I kept up karate training until I was about 20. Then I took a break for a few years and took up kung fu and yoga. I trained under many teachers, but it was my first yoga teacher, Rosemarie Holmes, who would constantly remind me that "breath is life. . . . it literally is." Around the same time I discovered Valda Moore, truly a world-class breathing teacher, who showed me many different ways to approach breathing and who inspired me to keep exploring the world of breath.

In my early twenties, I traveled to Europe and experienced a series of life-threatening and traumatic events. Apart from having all my luggage stolen and the threat of being attacked, I feared for my life one night when I was unexpectedly stranded on the streets of Rome. I used deep, calming breathing to help me cope with what could otherwise have been a mental breakdown. Through it all, I discovered a deep sense of inner peace and calm that I had never felt before. I was not used to this foreign feeling of inner peace but I liked it, and I wanted more of it. I realized that I could access this peaceful feeling only when I breathed in a certain way.

I was frustrated with the lack of information on practical breathing technique training in the West, so I decided to go straight to the experts and visit India on my way home to Australia.

While nobody can lay claim to the art of breathing as their own, in the East several thousand years ago, yogis, martial artists, t'ai chi masters, Tibetan monks, Taoists and others were exploring the breath. In fact, throughout the ages, sacred words have been used to describe the "breath of life," equating it with the spirit or life force—in India, they call it *prana;* in Latin, it was *spiritus;* in Ancient Greece, *pneuma;* in ancient Hawaii, *ha;* in China, *chi;* and Japan, *ki.* And while these ancient cultures did not know much about respiratory physiology, they believed that observation, awareness and the study of breath was the key to achieving physical, mental, emotional and spiritual mastery. Even today, breath continues to be explored as it was back then.

When I returned to Australia, I began working with the guests at Hippocrates Health Retreat in the Gold Coast hinterland. As I had no breathing teacher, I decided to put into practice everything I had learned up to that point. For the next two years, I lived in the mountains, ate healthy food and spent endless hours practicing deep breathing in the fresh mountain air. After a period of time, I began to experience a surge of boundless, vibrant energy. After sleeping no more than five hours, I would rise and run up and down mountains and not feel the slightest bit of fatigue! This went on day after day, and I felt absolutely great. The most amazing thing was that I continued to feel this boundless energy year after year.

I started giving lectures on breathing techniques at the retreat to help with exercise and for relaxation. People were enthusiastic and really interested in learning more about these methods of breathing. They wanted to learn how to breathe in all the different ways that I demonstrated.

Out of curiosity, I started asking people to show me their best and deepest breath, and I was intrigued by what I was constantly witnessing. I found that most people were able to demonstrate only a quick upper chest breath. Not many people could show me a really deep abdominal/diaphragmatic breath, despite the fact that they were trying really hard.

I felt that I needed to feel the difference between upper chest breathing compared with deep abdominal/diaphragmatic breathing. As an experiment, I decided to specifically practice upper chest breathing when exercising and for relaxation. I was astounded at the difference it made to my performance. I found I couldn't train or relax as effectively and generally didn't like the feeling it gave me, both mentally and physically. I resumed my abdominal/diaphragmatic breathing; I soon felt great again, and my performance improved. The experiment helped me to understand what everyone was experiencing with both shallow and deep breathing.

Word spread about this young girl in the mountains who was teaching breathing, and soon it seemed I was continuously checking people's breathing. People were coming from everywhere. I had offers to teach interstate and in New Zealand. I recall the first woman who offered to pay me to privately teach her various breathing techniques. I found it hard to believe that someone would want to pay me for doing something I found so natural!

I began to attract a lot of athletes and asthmatics. I also began receiving feedback on the benefits people gained once they began deep, good quality breathing. People kept asking me what I was doing to achieve such results. All I could say was that I showed them how to use their diaphragm and abdomen to breathe really deeply and to fill their lungs more than a standard survival breath. I also showed them a few breathing techniques that they could apply to different areas of their lifestyle.

Even after one session, people grasped the training enough to continue on by themselves. People I checked years later told me they were still able to use their improved breathing—especially for relaxation and exercise. Often just that one session was enough for them to grasp the fundamentals of good quality breathing.

Two years later I left Hippocrates and was hired by a center to teach a breathing course. For the first time, I had the chance to teach a variety of breathing techniques over an extended period of time. Around the same time, I also began working at the Golden Door Health Retreat, which had just opened. It was while I was at the Golden Door that I fine-tuned my whole approach to breathing training, and it was at this time that I developed the format for the breathing training session that I still use now. Many of the guests wanted to know more about the whole concept of breathing.

The management and staff at the Golden Door were also extremely supportive of my work and most of them took the time to do a breathing session with me.

After a few years of developing my breathing training and teaching, I had an offer to go to America and ended up working in a New York City dance studio. My time in New York was rewarding because my clients were so enthusiastic, and they found the breathing helped them perform better and cope with the stresses of big city life.

A year later, I returned home and with great enthusiasm resumed working once again at the Golden Door. The more people came to me wanting answers about breathing, the more I researched and observed breathing patterns.

Gradually, a few members of the medical profession started approaching me and asking me to privately train them. Some also asked me to help them with their patients who had particular breathing difficulties. I also began working with a couple of medical experts overseas to explore how different types of breathing can influence how we perform certain activities.

My inspiration for this book came when many adults demanded to know why information on something as important as the multidimensional aspects of breathing isn't given to us from an early age. My aim was to create an instructional and informative book on breathing. I've included techniques I have explored from the East as well as technical facts from physiologists and medical experts. I have also incorporated the feedback given to me by elite athletes as well as my clients.

Being of Greek origin, my dream was to write the book while overlooking the ocean on the Greek Islands. And that is exactly where I wrote it. I began on Santorini, my favorite place in the whole world, and finished it off on Syros and a few other islands. On my final day there, I sat, overlooking the beautiful Mediterranean Sea that had inspired me so much throughout the writing process, and I thought to myself: The gift of utilizing the breath was given to me. And now, with this book, I can finally give that gift back to anyone, anywhere and at any time. Yes, *dreams really do come true.*

Sophie Gabriel

For information on Sophie's Breathe for Life *video and audio tapes, breathing training courses and private breathing sessions, visit her website on **www.breatheforlife.com**. If you would like to contact Sophie, you can e-mail her at **sophie@breatheforlife.com**. Everyone will be answered, but please allow for possible delays of up to one month.*

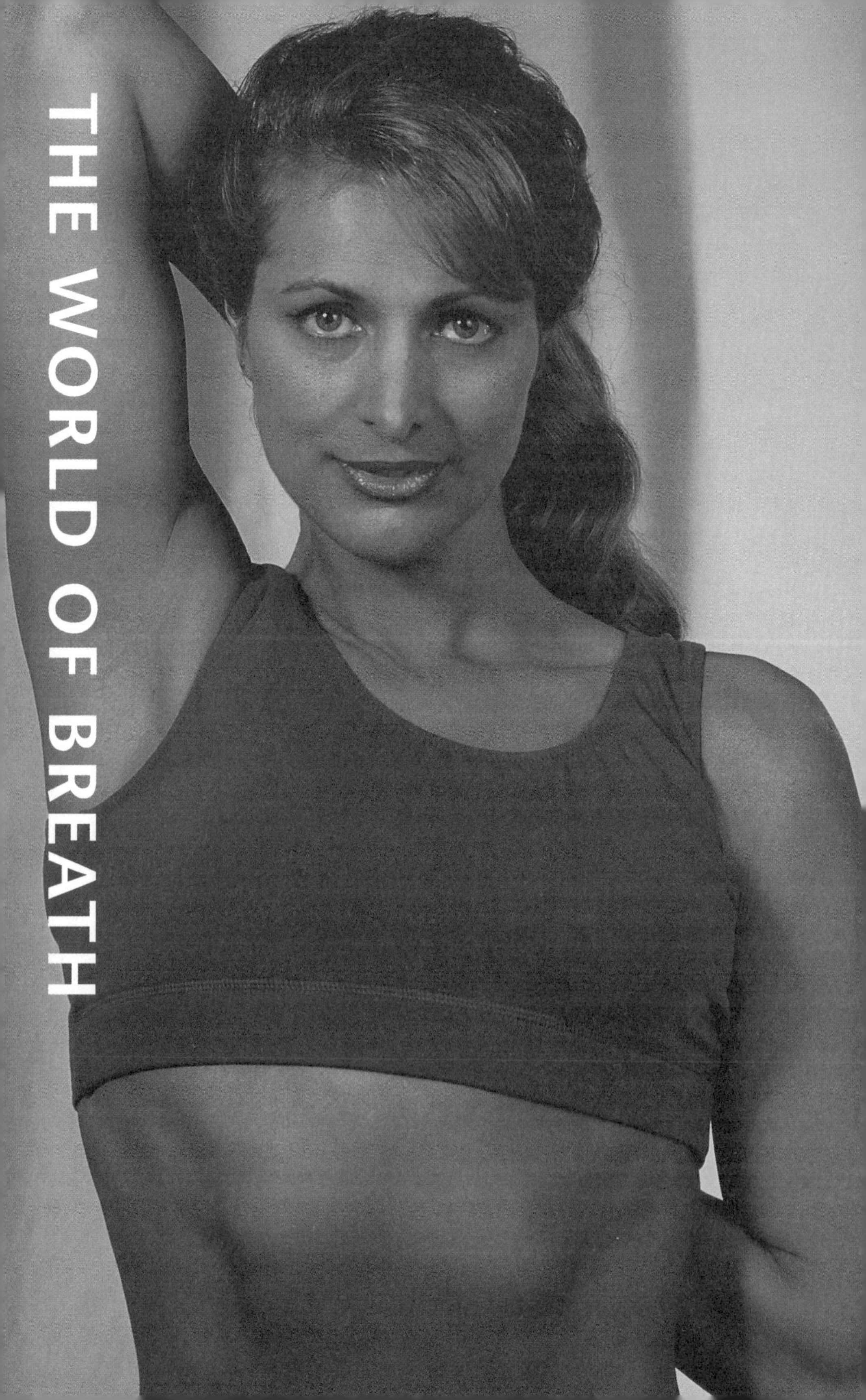

Welcome to the world of breath

"Why do I need to learn how to breathe? I breathe already, don't I?" This is a question I am constantly asked, and it is a valid one.

My response is this: Yes, of course we all breathe, but when I talk about breathing, I mean the "quality" of the breath, and the ability to be versatile with it. So let me ask you this: Can you breathe fully and deeply with ease? Are you able to appropriately adapt and control your breathing in any situation as your body's requirements change? Are you aware of the changes that occur to your body when you breathe a particular way? And have you experienced the dynamic effects of power breathing, or the calming effects of relaxation breathing?

I have spent the past 10 years examining the breathing habits and breathing quality of thousands of people—all sorts of people from all over the world. I have found that unless they have had some sort of breathing training, most people struggle to take a deep breath, and will admit to me that they don't know how. For many people, this inability to breathe fully can lead to shallow breathing. It seems that shallow, inappropriate breathing patterns are a common problem. Continually breathing in a faulty manner can lead to all sorts of health problems, as will be discussed later in greater detail.

The reasons why many of us have ended up with unhealthy breathing habits are complex. One of the main reasons is that we have simply developed bad habits as the years have gone by. Consider this—our breathing changes continually throughout the day, depending on what is demanded of us. For example, when we are stressed, such as after major surgery or traumatic experiences, our breathing becomes shallow; we tense up and occasionally hold our breath. Under normal circumstances, the breath would quickly return to normal. But if stress or fear is prolonged, the body may not have a chance to bounce back and shallow breathing can become habitual (because of the body's ability to adapt).

A couple of bad habits are poor posture and inflexibility leading to tightness of muscles in the chest and elsewhere. Add to that a lack of awareness and knowledge of how to utilize the multidimensional aspects of breathing techniques and you are left with an inability to breathe deeply, freely and with versatility.

Breath is life, and if you have been blocking the full potential of that life force over the years, how is it interfering with how you function as a whole being? The health industry is focused on what we eat and how we exercise. We are taught that "quality" of food is important—that we cannot continually eat processed food if we expect to maintain a high level of health. But do we stop to consider the "quality" of our breathing? How many of us know if our style of breathing is healthy or not?

You might suggest that exercise is all you need to develop healthy breathing. Exercise is essential, of course, but do you breathe correctly and appropriately for each sport/exercise you participate in? And did you know that there are ways in which you can develop the breath that will have positive affects on your health, as well as increasing your ability to exercise?

I describe specialized breathing exercises and techniques as "internal breathing training." When physical exercise ("external breathing training") is combined with internal breathing exercises (see pages 31–32), you have a perfect combination that guarantees a total workout for the whole respiratory system, which improves the oxygen-carbon-dioxide exchange function of the respiratory system.

Many people, particularly those with serious breathing problems, doubt that it is possible to unlearn bad breathing habits. Yet, time and time again, I have witnessed thousands of people's breathing improve, regardless of their initial manner of breathing.

The purpose of this book is to show you how to reestablish quality breathing and independently improve and maintain healthy breathing habits throughout your life. The fact is, no matter who you are or what you do, learning how to breathe fully, without any inhibitions or constraints, will enhance the quality of your life.

Being able to take full, deep breaths without any inhibitions is a way of internally relaxing and revitalizing your body and mind. My greatest wish for you is that you will learn how to breathe fully so you can recapture that endless, childlike energy and enthusiasm for life that lies within us all.

What is a good quality breath?

I began observing how people breathe in a variety of different circumstances. I have also personally examined the breathing pattern of people from different backgrounds, nationalities and ages. Some of my clients have had respiratory problems, such as asthma or a missing lung, while others have been experienced singers or elite/professional athletes. In between those two extremes, I have worked with all sorts of different people who, for whatever reason, wanted to improve their breathing.

In order to assess the quality of how a person breathes, I ask them to demonstrate their best quality breath, and to make it their longest and deepest. After a few breaths, I time how long the person can inhale, and do the same for their exhalation. I also carefully watch *how* they breathe. When I ask them to demonstrate their best quality breath, I have observed that there is a common way most people breathe, and that there is an obvious difference between people who have had some form of good quality breathing training and those who have not.

With *good quality breathing,* the diaphragm is the main muscle used, along with the intercostal muscles (muscles between the ribs). There is no exaggerated movement of the upper chest, sternum and shoulders. Correct, deep, diaphragmatic breathing utilizes the entire lung capacity. Deep breathing means to breathe fully, resulting in full expansion of the thorax vertically, sideways, front and back. A full breath executed properly is performed in a relaxed manner without strain, struggle or force.

A *poor quality breath* is shallow, erratic, lacks rhythm and is insufficient for optimum health. Shallow breathing often expands only the sternum and upper chest. Therefore, predominately using the upper chest and shoulder muscles to breathe in and out does not utilize the *full* strength of the diaphragm, which results in a limited amount of air entering the lungs. Not only does this cause a reduced amount of ventilation, but continuously breathing in this way can lead to fatigue. Poor quality or forceful breathing can also produce tightness in the chest, diaphragm and abdominal area. The rib cage tends to be notably restricted—it is unable to move fully and freely as it would when entirely flexible.

When trying to produce a good quality breath, I have observed that people who have had no previous breathing training breathe mainly in and out of their upper chest. It is usually a quick, shallow and abrupt breath with a lifting of the chest and shoulders. With exhalation, the breath is slightly longer and there is a sinking of the chest and dropping of the shoulders. People often struggle to try and breathe in and out as much as they can, with an exaggerated use of the upper chest and little ability to breathe deeply no matter how hard they try. Even with numerous attempts to increase the depth and duration, the results are the same.

People who have had some sort of specialized breathing training display much better quality breathing than those who haven't. Some of these include singers, athletes, actors, divers, musicians who play wind instruments (including Australia's own Aboriginal didgeridoo players), and students of meditation, relaxation, yoga, t'ai chi, martial arts, and also certain forms of bodywork such as Feldenkrais, the Alexander Technique and Pilates. When they are initially asked for their best quality breath, in most cases, the exhalation is of a high standard. There is no unnecessary movement of the upper chest, and there is clear indication of good use of the diaphragm. Their diaphragms are strong, toned and flexible. However, when they were consciously demonstrating their best breath, there was a notable difference between their exhalation and their inhalation.

After carefully observing the inhalation and comparing it with the exhalation, the person notices that the inhalation is always shorter and weaker; the exhalation is typically longer and stronger. I am often asked why and I will explain it in greater detail later. But for now, if you consider the nature of most breathing training, it is the exhalation that is often more developed.

Let's look at singing as an example. Singers have learned how to control their breathing and to release a lengthy, good quality exhalation in order to sing properly. Inhalation, on the other hand, does not need to be developed to the same extent. But singers who have asked me to help them with their whole manner of breathing found that they were able to pull in more breath between notes. Consequently, this helps them to sing better and eliminates the uncomfortable and restrictive feeling they often experienced when they were required to inhale.

I have also worked with quite a few athletes over the years. They are a distinct group to work with and my approach with them is entirely different. Interestingly enough, when I asked them to demonstrate particular ways of breathing, such as for flexibility exercises, they usually didn't know how. However, once they learned how to consciously use and efficiently control their diaphragm, they became top quality "versatile" breathers. They are able to breathe extremely well in a number of different ways, both for the inhalation and exhalation; their quality, duration, power and ability to control the breath is excellent once the basic principles are mastered. In fact, it has been my observation that athletes show more overall improvement in the end than any other group with whom I have worked.

There are two reasons for this. First, basic breathing during exercise demands that athletes regulate the breath and take in and expel voluminous amounts of air. Second, as a result of exercise, the diaphragm is powerfully strengthened. When I show athletes how to use the diaphragm specifically to control their breathing, they have a big advantage over most people because of their huge lung capacity, the extra strength of their diaphragm and their ability to regulate the breath. I show them how to maximize and utilize their diaphragm, and how to take in a large breath both when they are resting and while they are exercising. They are also taught how to apply particular breathing techniques to their training.

What happens when I breathe shallowly?

When you breathe in a shallow manner, predominately using your upper chest, sternum and shoulder muscles, a reduced amount of air enters the lungs—the practice of upper chest breathing does not allow total inflation of the lungs. It is likely you will have limited breathing capacity if you continue to breathe in a restricted and shallow manner, since the body has the ability to adapt.

If shallow breathing becomes habitual, it can create a state of unease and anxiety. It is the most exhausting and stressful way to breathe, requiring a greater amount of effort and producing the least benefits.

Occasional upper chest breathing occurs as a natural response to dangerous or stressful situations. The problem lies in the unconscious continual use of shallow, upper chest breathing, which can negatively influence our physical and mental health.

Why should I learn to breathe fully?

If you were dying of thirst in a desert and you came across two glasses of water—one full and the other only a third full—which would you choose? Naturally, the full one, but if you continually breathe in a shallow manner and never do any form of deep breathing, it is the same as reaching for the less full glass when your body would obviously function better on the full one.

It's such a pity to see people who are imprisoned in their own bodies, who want to be able to breathe better but are unable to take a full, deep and satisfying breath. Why should anyone have to struggle to do something that should be effortless? Breathing fully is our birthright.

If you cannot breathe deeply without effort . . . why not? Why are you unable to take a full breath without strain and struggle? Do you want to accept as a way of life this struggle to fully breathe? If you knew you could do something about it, would you? You can improve your breathing. Once you do, I know you will never want to go back to your old ways of stressful and limited shallow breathing.

After a person experiences their first deep, uninhibited breath, it becomes obvious to them that breathing deeply is not just about the mere unconscious act of breathing in and out. I have found that once a person feels the difference between shallow and full breathing, their whole attitude changes. I constantly witness the excitement people feel when they "break through" and experience freedom in their breathing. Once you learn to consciously breathe deeply, you will have to expend less effort with any kind of breathing you do.

If you have poor breathing habits, you will still be able to exercise. But the breathing required for exercise is not the same as that taught in a breathing training session. If you know you need to improve the standard of your breathing, I advise you to work on that separately and learn healthy breathing habits. When you feel ready, you should also increase your breathing capacity by exercising. Once you learn good quality breathing, you won't revert back to your inappropriate breathing patterns, even when you are not exercising.

The positive benefits of deep breathing

When you breathe deeply, powerfully and proficiently, you will see results on a number of levels. Physically it will help you to:

- build and develop a solid foundation for healthy breathing without exhausting the body (as with some forms of exercise).
- tone all the muscles involved in respiration.
- easily perform physical activities, including sports.
- improve your general health (your internal organs are nourished with oxygen).
- expand and contract your rib cage with ease.
- release accumulated tension, allowing you to relax more easily.
- rest and feel refreshed.
- subdue physical pain (e.g., during childbirth and while exercising).
- strengthen and revitalize your nervous system (by decreasing stress and increasing feelings of well-being).

Deep breathing ensures that an ample supply of air reaches its way through the lungs. Also, air sacs that have previously been partially ventilated, as a result of shallow breathing, are now aerated, increasing your capacity to nourish the blood with oxygen.

On a mental level, you will find that deep, rhythmical breathing creates a harmonious emotional state. You will feel calmer and more relaxed, deal with stress better, and feel more centered and focused. Many people complain that they are either hyped up and functioning on nervous energy, or they barely have enough energy to get by and feel lethargic most of the time. Paradoxically, deep breathing can be very invigorating and calming at the same time.

Once you start breathing fully, simultaneously increasing your levels of exercise and improving your eating habits, you can expect to see your energy levels soar. You will sleep better, wake up refreshed and feel an increase of energy. The spark of life that may have been dim is all of a sudden lit . . . and you will want to move and get more out of life!

The causes of faulty and shallow breathing

People often ask me why their breathing has become weakened or less than ideal. There are many reasons. As explained in the introduction, this book will be referring only to the average healthy person whose lifestyle habits influence the manner in which they breathe. As babies, we breathe without inhibition, the way nature intended. Unfortunately, unless our breathing is continually developed, we tend to lose the ability to breathe fully and powerfully. Why?

Let's start at the very beginning . . . our first breath! Does our very first breath have any influence on how we breathe later in life? Most people don't believe so. However, one well-known French obstetrician thinks it does. In his book *Birth Without Violence*, Frederick Le Boyer presents a number of his controversial views on how a baby should be born, including how newborn babies should take their first breath.

Babies practice breathing before they are born. When a baby has just emerged from the womb and is still attached to the umbilical cord, one of its next major tasks is to take its first breath outside of its mother's womb without the cord. Le Boyer states that cutting the cord before the baby is ready to breathe on its own causes an abrupt gasp for the first breath, which lays the foundation for problems with breathing later in life. He believes that the cord should not be cut until it stops pulsing. This results in the baby's taking a relaxed first breath, without any stress or panic.

Of course many of you would disagree with Le Boyer's theories and concepts. Interestingly enough, I have had numerous mothers report to me (in Australia) that their babies were immediately placed on their chest after birth, and the cord was not immediately cut (the times varied).

Babies breathe with a relaxed abdomen and change their breathing in a fluid manner. By the time they start school, signs of breathing problems are beginning to show, as is evidenced by the alarmingly high incidence of asthma in young children. Sometimes, children having tantrums make a habit of holding their breath, resulting in poor breathing at a very early age. But the significant difference with children is that they naturally adjust their breathing for every activity, whereas adults are not as instinctive. So generally, children tend to breathe relatively well in their early years. It would be ideal to teach all children at this stage to become aware of and maintain good quality breathing habits, and to train them to develop their breathing capabilities further.

During the challenging teenage years, the first signs of poor breathing habits are more obvious. There is so much to deal with emotionally, and it is common and typical to respond to emotional confusion by holding our breath. In addition to dealing with the stress of growing up, there is the added stress of studying and examinations. Consequently, poor posture sets in as we slouch over our desks to study and sit in unnatural poses at computers for hours. It is becoming apparent that the youth of today, on average, are not as fit and do not have the breathing capacity of their grandparents. Is it any wonder that, even at this youthful age, so many young people complain about feeling tired and becoming breathless easily?

As we progress into adulthood, we take our poor breathing habits with us. Unfortunately, without corrective breathing training, these habits can unconsciously become ingrained. Unless people are fit, by the time most are elderly, their ability to breathe deeply and powerfully has decreased. Many elderly people find it a struggle to breathe and can become breathless even when performing simple everyday tasks. When I ask them to take their deepest breath, the result is often a lifeless gasp. As we age, our rib cage stiffens, we tend to exercise less and are generally not as active as we were in our youth. Is it any wonder that our breathing becomes so much weaker as we grow older? Breathing training is therefore very important as we age.

So you can see the progression. Habitual, shallow breathing does not just happen (unless the problem is due to disease). It is a result of years of neglect and years of failing to deal adequately with any of the following factors.

Stress

We are all faced with stress in our lives, and our inability to cope with it effectively is one of the most common problems we face today. Not all stress is bad for us. Stress can help us push ahead and get things done; it can make us more productive. However, being in an overly stressed state for too long a period can have a detrimental effect, mentally and physically. We can become so stressed that we can hardly breathe. Instead of allowing enough time for our breathing to return to normal, we become anxious about all that we have to say and do; as a result our breathing stays shallow and the vicious cycle continues. This can cause our overall breathing patterns to be thrown out of balance.

Ongoing stress creates bad breathing habits that can become permanent unless consciously changed. These have a negative effect on our breathing. Accumulated anger, anxiety, depression, frustration and other negative emotions interfere with healthy breathing. Learning how to diffuse and cope with overwhelming emotions can help you avoid this problem, making it easier for you to cope with a high level of stress and recuperate properly.

Poor posture, muscular tension and "rigid rib cages"

Most tension is a result of prolonged muscle contraction, poor posture and lack of flexibility. The negative effects that muscular tension and poor posture have on breathing cannot be overstated. A sunken chest and drooping shoulders stop us from breathing fully and freely. Any excess tension in the face, neck, throat, shoulders and respiratory muscles will constrain deep breathing and can result in habitual shallow breathing. In particular, if the muscles around the chest and rib cage area are inflexible and tight, you will feel uncomfortable and your breathing will be restricted.

Also, the inability to move the ribs inward and outward can constrain full breathing. As children, everyone can move their rib cages with ease and fluidity. As adults, our rib cage tends to become stiff as a natural consequence of aging and lack of use. I call it the "rigid rib cage syndrome." Unfortunately, it does not take long to become inflexible. From the time we are young, all the muscles of the body gradually begin to lose their natural flexibility if they are not regularly stretched.

Habitual tightening of the abdominal muscles and the inability to let go of that tension is another cause of constrained breathing. However, flexibility and correct posture allow the diaphragm and abdomen to move freely and in harmony.

When we learn to efficiently use the full range of movement that our chest wall and rib cage is capable of, we can fully ventilate the lungs and give them a thorough workout. However, most people have no idea how to do this unless they are shown during specific kinds of breathing training.

Lack of exercise

Everyone is aware of the importance of exercise. A sedentary lifestyle will reduce your fitness and breathing capacity. We live in a society that has machinery to accommodate many tasks in our everyday life. There is very little body movement required in a normal day compared with 50 years ago. So we miss out on daily activities that would naturally cause us to move about and breathe more. If you exercise regularly, you compensate for this lack of movement. If you do not exercise, then your lungs and respiratory muscles will lose both natural elasticity and strength respectively.

Your occupation can affect your breathing. It may be that you are often overstressed and under pressure. You may be required to lean over a desk for most of the day, which automatically limits your full range of breathing and eventually leads to poor quality posture.

If you do not exercise and you have a job that requires you to sit for most of the day, your respiratory system will not get an adequate workout for a basic level of health. Poor quality air caused by heating, air conditioners and lack of sufficient ventilation can affect the airways. Compare this kind of occupation with that of a snow ski instructor who is outside in the fresh air, moving about constantly, stretching and lifting. Sedentary office workers should compensate by making it a priority to exercise regularly. Deep breathing and proper posture can help to counteract negative effects.

At the extreme end of the problem, it could be that you are constantly inhaling chemical fumes, such as solvents used in paints, or particles that are hazardous to your lungs, such as asbestos.

It is standard practice now to have safety equipment available for most hazardous jobs involving dangerous fumes and damaging particles. If you know your occupation can cause problems to your respiratory system and you feel you need better quality protective equipment, perhaps you could discuss the matter with your manager or supervisor. If you ever meet someone who has developed a respiratory disease as a result of a hazardous job, I believe you will feel it well worthwhile to make any effort to prevent having the same problem.

Smoke

It is a well-documented fact, and all of us know by now, that smoking causes damage to your lungs, leading to chronic bronchitis, emphysema and lung cancer. Breathing patterns caused by these organic diseases unfortunately cannot be reversed by breathing training. These serious conditions need to be treated medically. A couple of the numerous negative effects of smoking are a dramatic reduction to your breathing capacity and a decrease of the oxygen-carrying capacity of the blood.

Pollution

Think of what it is like when you are in the country, and how you naturally draw in the fresh air as deeply as you can. Now think about what it is like when you are in a polluted area. Pollution can directly damage your airways and lungs so you tend to instinctively decrease your breathing, which is the body's way of rejecting anything that may harm it.

Genetic weakness

If you have always had problems with your breathing, and if your respiratory system is the first to suffer when you become run down, then perhaps it is your genetic weakness. It depends on the cause and your constitution as to whether or not your conditions will worsen as you age. But whatever your problem, it is worth learning as much as you can about how to keep your respiratory system strong and healthy. If you can accept the fact that you will need to take extra care and be vigilant about looking after it for the rest of your life, you have at least done your best to prevent problems occurring as a result of neglect. (As always, I recommend you take advice from your doctor or specialist about these matters.)

Food

For people such as athletes, singers and public speakers, an efficient use of abdominal/diaphragmatic breathing is important (see page 35). Abdominal muscles are overstretched when we eat too much; therefore, the diaphragm cannot work as efficiently. Remember how it feels after you have eaten a huge holiday dinner and how you can barely breathe? Eating too much (heavy) food is inadvisable when you need to breathe deeply for a particular purpose.

Some people find they are allergic to particular milk. Not everyone reacts the same way. Most people can tolerate anything, but some people are more sensitive than others and have a food intolerance. For example, if your body reacts as a result of drinking too much milk, then cut down or switch to a non-dairy milk. If you know you have a problem, I suggest you experiment to see what is best for you.

Clothes

Restrictive clothing can interfere with our breathing. Women in particular impede their full range of breath when they wear belts and certain clothes that are obviously too tight, limiting the natural movement of the abdomen. If you have a problem with your breathing due to restrictive clothing, you may need to loosen your tie or let out your belt a notch or two when driving or sitting. Or you might consider wearing something that allows you to breathe more comfortably.

Pain, illness and injury

Any physical pain, illness or injury can cause the breath to change in order to cope—this is a normal response. There is a natural tendency to hold our breath when we are in pain. The best advice I can give you is to allow the body to breathe in a way that feels the most appropriate to cope with the pain or discomfort. One of the best ways to relax is to abdominally breathe, breathing deep, slow breaths. This may help to subdue the pain and make you feel better. This form of breathing is encouraged at childbirth to reduce labor pain. Any problems that are chronic or prolonged may lead to shallow breathing that may become a life-long problem.

Traumatic incidents, for example surgery, death of a loved one, motor accidents and other events that lead to emotional burden and fear, are incidents that trigger "psychogenic" (of mental origin) shallow breathing. Please refer to the chapter Coping with pain (page 146) for more detail.

Training the breath

Dr. Gay Hendricks is a U.S. physician who has been measuring people's breathing capacity on a simple machine called the Voldyne for the last 10 years. When he began this work, his own breathing was at the normal capacity for his age. Ten years later, his capacity is equal to that of a 19-year-old. Why? In one of his books, he states that it's because he has been specifically training his breath.

There is a physiological reason why it is possible to change and improve our breathing. Breathing is an involuntary and automatic self-regulating function of the nervous system. This means that our breathing will continue to keep us alive without any conscious effort on our part. It is also a part of the voluntary nervous system, and interestingly, breathing is a function we can consciously change at will. Thus, as a result of our conscious or habitual behavior, we can alter our breathing in a positive or negative way.

Breathing is a mechanism of the body that adapts to change and, by its very nature, changes often. Our breathing can change instantly because of a movement, a thought, or an emotion of any kind, particularly intense ones.

All the other involuntary functions, such as digestion and circulation, will continue no matter how much we try to stop the process. For example, we cannot eat some food and consciously stop the digestion of it halfway. But we can take in a breath and stop halfway if we wish. We can also lengthen the breath out and purposely change it if our activity requires a particular kind of breath, such as for exercise or singing.

Breathing training teaches us to control our breathing and change it whenever we need to. It also teaches us to expand our lung capacity by consciously increasing our breath size. This gives us the opportunity to be flexible and versatile in every aspect of our breathing.

The techniques and exercises outlined in the section Practical training are designed to develop, fine-tune and improve your general breathing ability. Breathing training programs can be designed according to your personal needs. Each sport, for instance, has a particular breathing program that is tailor-made for it. Another person can design a program to improve specific breathing needs or weaknesses, such as strengthening inspiratory muscles.

The best way to learn about breathing training is with a teacher or coach. However, breathing teachers are few and far between. I mean, have you ever found one in the Yellow Pages? This book has been produced to make up for that absence. No instructor would ever recommend a book over personal training, and I do not either. I do not claim that you will achieve the same results as you would with an instructor, but I do believe you can learn enough from this book to improve your general breathing ability. The instructions I give here are the exact instructions I would give you in a private training session. How much and how quickly you improve depends on the effort you put into learning. Other influential factors include whether you have had any breathing training at all; if you have a genetic weakness of the respiratory system; your posture; your job; whether you exercise; how motivated you are to learn; and how much you absorb.

Basic breathing training—what to expect

When you begin formal breathing training, you are taught to breathe properly using healthy breathing habits, both for inhalation and exhalation, and to accurately learn how to fully use the diaphragm. You also learn a number of different breathing techniques. Bad habits that interfere with healthy breathing are eliminated, and good habits are encouraged. You are taught to become aware of the difference between correct and incorrect breathing habits.

The most common problem I see when people begin breathing training is the inability to take a long, deep relaxing breath, or a really powerful one. This means their ability to be versatile with their breathing is limited, making it difficult for them to relax fully or exert themselves during a strenuous task, such as exercise.

Awareness is a crucial component of basic breathing training. You need to become aware of the habits that prevent you from breathing healthily. As the body innately knows how to breathe perfectly, if you have a problem with your breathing, it is a matter of "un-learning" what has interrupted the natural flow of the breath. Think of it as a realignment to bring every aspect of your breathing back to the harmonious function that nature intended it to be.

Corrective breathing training requires you to be still while you closely and consciously observe the quality of your breath. This way, you can fully focus and begin to notice unhealthy breathing habits. Once you are aware of your improper habits, you can begin to correct them and to focus on improving your ideal breathing habits. Proper breathing training also aims to make inhalation as good, in terms of quality, strength and length, as exhalation.

If your incorrect breathing habits have become ingrained over a long period of time, you will need perseverance and patience. But if you persist and continue to practice good quality breathing habits, you will feel the positive changes.

By focusing your mind and breath, and by specifically controlling the diaphragm, you can breathe as deeply as possible. The upper and the base of the lungs are filled by the abdominal/diaphragmatic breath.

Once you master the basic breathing training, you will function much more efficiently with any type of breathing that you do. You will be able to control your breathing for different activities in order to breathe:

- slower
- quicker
- powerfully
- softer
- longer
- shorter
- deeper

So for all the activities that life demands, you can learn to adjust your breathing and function to the best of your ability.

In summary, basic breathing training will help you achieve the following:

- Inhalation is developed to be as good (or almost as good) as exhalation in quality and duration.
- All the muscles involved in respiration are greatly strengthened—especially the diaphragm.
- Flexibility is increased for all the muscles involved in respiration and the whole rib cage.
- Ribs open up and become noticeably movable, inward and outward.
- Basic proper posture is adapted, especially if chest is habitually sunken and shoulders droop forward, constraining the breath.

Developing your breathing

Once our breathing has improved to a certain level via basic breathing training, an on-going training program must be adopted to maintain the benefits and to prevent the weakening of the respiratory system that is a natural consequence of aging.

If you want to keep your whole respiratory system in basic good health, then for as long as you live you will need to exercise and challenge your breathing. You cannot maintain a healthy functioning respiratory system by practicing breathing exercises and/or physical exercise for a period of time and then stopping. Some form of daily exercise for the lungs is commonly recommended to keep toning them and to prevent them from weakening in old age.

How much time you should spend on breathing training will depend on your goals. Obviously professional athletes or singers need to work at their breathing daily. For others, a 20-minute walk every day might be enough for their level of fitness and health.

Internal breathing training can help those people who do not exercise because of pain or disability and those who simply don't want to exercise. While it cannot replace exercise, it can at least compensate by actively working your breath. Those people who do like to exercise, but struggle with it, will find that they will be able to exercise without becoming so breathless. Their general fitness levels can gradually increase and improve. Even athletes have found a faster rate in recovery, increased focus and improved overall flexibility after taking part in a specialized breathing training program.

A firm commitment to whatever program suits you best is the important thing. (Even if you cannot exercise, you can still follow a program that includes breathing exercises.) Once you start, you will begin to lay the foundation for an overall healthy manner of breathing. Whatever time and effort you put in, you will gain back tenfold.

Automatic and conscious breathing

I am often asked, "What is the best way to breathe?" The answer is paradoxical: there is no one best way to breathe because your breathing requirements change with different circumstances; and there are better ways of breathing for everything that you do.

It is important to be able to change your breathing according to the demand. Sometimes a full breath is needed; other times, a gentle one. Once you begin to understand this, you are on your way to becoming what I call an "ideal breather." Whether you breathe appropriately or not in different circumstances could positively or negatively affect your health, energy, emotional state and general performance. Breathing appropriately refers to both natural and conscious breathing.

There are times when a change in your breathing should happen spontaneously, such as in response to emotions. There are other times when you may need to consciously change your breathing pattern, for example, blowing out a candle. When referring to good quality conscious breathing, there are specific methods that achieve optimum results—for example, deep abdominal breathing as opposed to upper chest breathing for relaxation.

Automatic breathing

There are two kinds of breathing that occur automatically: natural breathing and self-regulating responses.

First, we will take a look at natural breathing, which I also refer to as "survival" and "quiet" breathing. It is the breathing that takes place automatically, continually and spontaneously; the breathing that keeps us alive and functioning.

Natural breathing

While it is difficult to accurately assess how you breathe naturally, you may gain a few insights by asking yourself whether you breathe in with your nose or mouth, and whether you breathe out with your nose or mouth.

If you breathe through your mouth, ask yourself why? Is it because you feel it is the only way you can breathe sufficiently in comfort?

You should also consider whether:

- you breathe in and out from your chest or abdomen
- your breath is abrupt or erratic
- your breathing is audible
- you do any of the following on a regular basis:
  - ‡ struggle to take a normal breath
  - ‡ experience a constant tightness in the chest that makes you feel that your breathing is inhibited.

These are indications of shallow breathing. Do you feel that you are a shallow breather? If so, is it only in certain circumstances or is it a constant way of breathing?

Do the following descriptions match the way you breathe?

- Your breathing is deep, rhythmical and flowing freely.
- You know exactly what kind of breath is needed for each function that you do.
- Your breathing changes appropriately as your activities do.
- Your neck, shoulders, face, chest and abdomen are comfortable and relaxed.
- Your breathing feels harmonious and effortless.

These are indications of proper breathing. Do you feel you are a "good quality" breather?

TESTING YOUR NATURAL BREATHING AT REST

This is a test to count how many times you (naturally) breathe per minute. The most effective way is to get someone to count for you. If this is not possible, you may count by yourself but the results may not be as accurate. Either way, it is important that you or the other person simply observe what is happening during this test. You should not try to deliberately change the way that you breathe or the results will be invalid. Using an inhalation and exhalation as one breath, count how many times you breathe per minute for two minutes. Then divide your result in half to get an average, and write the amount down. If your score is above 15, it is important to immediately see your doctor. Breathing 16 times per minute or more while you are resting is a sign of shallow breathing and could indicate early signs of a disease or health problem. Adults who habitually breathe in a healthy and relaxed manner breathe about 10 to 12 breaths per minute. (Children naturally breathe a lot faster.) When I ask for a show of hands from my audience, on average, I find adults normally breathe around 14 to 16 times per minute when resting. However, when adults are stressed, there is an increase to 20 or more breaths per minute. Take a moment to consider the answer to all the questions above, and assess yourself on your opinion of your natural breathing. Do you feel it is functioning optimally, or do you detect certain habits that are perhaps interfering with the ideal functioning of your natural breathing? There are four stages to a complete breath:

1. inhalation
2. transition from inhalation to exhalation
3. exhalation
4. transition from exhalation to inhalation (an expiratory pause)

Ideally, each stage gently blends into the other without any abruptness. The transitions between breaths are an important component in healthy breathing. They help to give a harmonious rhythm and keep your mind and body relaxed. Depending on the type of breathing, the time of the transition will vary, and the one after the exhalation is commonly the shortest. Sometimes transitions will happen too quickly or inharmoniously, indicating uncoordinated breathing. Other times, transitions will be a lot longer, such as when you are deeply relaxed. But for basic healthy breathing, there should be a natural, full completion of the four stages. Following is a checklist of "healthy" and "distressed" breathing traits.

Healthy natural breathing

- Breathing occurs in and out of the nose only.
- There is a slow, rhythmical movement of the abdomen, with no exaggerated movement of the upper chest or shoulders.
- The breath is inaudible.
- The breath appears relaxed and effortless with no sign of strain, gasping or struggle.
- All four stages of breathing happen very gently and blend into one another without any abruptness.

Signs of "respiratory distress"

- Breathing predominately into and out of the upper chest.
- Lifting shoulders and/or upper chest to breathe in (as in some severe respiratory conditions).
- Dropping shoulders and/or upper chest to exhale.
- Breath is quick and shallow.
- Whole manner of breathing is erratic and has no rhythm.
- There is an inconsistent transition period between inhalation and exhalation.
- Audible sound of sniffing, sighing, puffing or gasping.
- Breathing is constantly an effort, and it is a struggle to breathe in and/or out.

Self-regulating responses/reflex controls

The body is designed to automatically respond in various ways (yawning, sneezing, sighing, etc.) when it needs a change in breathing either on the inhalation and/or the exhalation. The body, in its wisdom, always adapts to whatever demands are being placed upon it by making you breathe in a specific way to bring it back into balance. For example, a yawn causes the lungs to stretch thereby increasing oxygen to your lungs.

The manner of breathing for self-regulating responses may recruit the mouth, as this is the body's way of drawing in or expelling a large amount of breath instantly. Everyone requires a big breath every so many breaths. Yawning or sighing, for example, are a normal part of breathing.

There are also self-regulating responses to emotional situations, such as laughing and crying, in addition to responses to what is considered an urgent or dangerous situation. For example, you cough in order to expel a foreign object from your body. Gasping and suspending the breath are used in intense moments, such as when you are about to have a car accident. By suspending your breath, you can concentrate with maximum focus on the best way to handle the situation—whether to slam on the breaks or swerve to the side.

We are all familiar with the term "fight or flight." It is a response that automatically happens as soon as you are alerted to danger. A whole series of physiological and psychological changes takes place during this response. It is the brain that stimulates the changes, one being a release of adrenaline from the adrenal glands. The brain controls the release of adrenaline and this produces a number of changes, including enlarging the airways to allow more effective breathing. Other examples of these changes are an increase in alertness as well as in the rate and force of the heart's beating.

But you do not need to be in danger for the body to react. Any form of anxiety, such as stress or anger, puts the body into an "alerted" state, in varying degrees, depending on the circumstance and intensity of the emotion.

Do you find yourself *yawning* when you are tired or bored? The true cause of yawning is debatable; it has been said to occur as a result of physiological as well as psychological reasons. Whatever the reason, when your breathing decreases, it subsequently decreases the body's supply of oxygen. A yawn is one example of how the body increases oxygen, which is why you might need to yawn more than once until the task has been achieved. When performed properly, a yawn is a good quality breath. The breath is taken deep into the lungs and the ribs fully expand. Then there is a period of time when the inhalation is slowly changing over to the exhalation, which also is deeper than normal.

This kind of deep, full breath allows ease of stretch of the lungs through the secretion of an important substance called "surfactant." In turn, the oxygen brought in by the deep, full breath helps to improve circulation, making you feel more awake. Also, the facial muscles relax and tension from the shoulders and neck is eased. This is why it is not a good idea to stifle a yawn. When you can, allow yourself to stretch out completely, open your mouth and allow the body to fully yawn as much as it needs and wants to. When a yawn is executed properly, even if it takes a few times, you should notice your breathing has improved and that you feel slightly more alert.

Sighing is another common habit, particularly for shallow breathers, who tend to sigh more than normal. It is often caused by emotional stress. If you are sighing excessively, this is a sign that the body is deprived of deep breathing and your breathing has become shallow. The bodily action of sighing counteracts shallow, upper chest breathing, and it is the body's way of indicating that a deep method of breathing is required. So if you are sighing a lot, do not stop yourself from sighing as much as you need to, but be aware that you might have formed the habit of sighing or your body is indicating that your breathing needs to deepen. To remedy the problem, you will need to somehow increase your depth of breathing. I suggest you do some deep breathing exercises, and if you can, some general exercise. Even a 20-minute walk each day can do wonders to increase your breathing capacity.

Coughing and sneezing both clear out your nose, throat and airways of any irritations, food or foreign objects. This protects the lungs from harm and prevents obstructions in your respiratory passage.

Conscious breathing

As the name suggests, conscious breathing refers to the type of breathing that we deliberately control. Once you understand how to control and manipulate your breathing patterns, you will be able to breathe for specific situations and results. Good examples of this are breathing for running, relaxation, and lifting a heavy object.

TESTING YOUR CONSCIOUS BREATHING AT REST

Examining your ability to breathe consciously is a good way to assess your breathing habits. First, take the best quality breath that you can—as long and deep as possible. Note whether you breathed in and out of your nose or mouth. If it was through the mouth, is that because it is the only way you can take a deep breath? Unless it is impossible for you to do so, for the rest of the exercise, breathe in and out of your nose only, even if you feel more comfortable breathing through your mouth.

Next we will time how long you can breathe in and out. (Note: you must count the breath for as long as you hear sound, rather than by movement of the chest or shoulders.) So with the mouth closed, breathe in for as long as you can and time it. Next, time your longest and deepest exhalation.

Try this two or three times and work out your average. I suggest you write down this initial timing so that later you can see how you have progressed.

Is your exhalation much longer and/or stronger than your inhalation? Do you find it more difficult to inhale rather than exhale? Write down what you observe.

If you are experienced in any form of good quality breathing training, the ideal breath is to have the inhalation as good as your exhalation. A consistent, good quality inhalation and exhalation that are equally as strong show excellent breath control and are easily reached when you are proficient with your breathing skills.

Once again, take a few of your best quality breaths in and out of the nose only, and note what area expands: the upper chest or the abdomen area? If it is the upper chest, can you breathe predominately using your diaphragm and do so without obviously moving your upper chest? If not, why not? Is it because you find it a struggle? Is it confusing or just not possible?

Now that you have read the first section of the book, you are aware that different kinds of breathing are required for different kinds of situations. But do you know how to properly change your breathing according to each demand? Do you know how to breathe to relax? For power and strength? To focus or to concentrate? To fully move your rib cage? To control specific parts of your respiratory system so that you have total control over how you breathe in any given circumstance?

Ask yourself whether you experience any of the following:

- excessive yawning and sighing
- continuous holding of your breath
- habitual shallow breathing into the upper chest
- lifting and dropping the upper chest and shoulders
- not breathing properly with bodily movements
- abdominal muscles are habitually tensed and you are unable to consciously relax them
- forcing the breath with too much unnecessary strain
- struggling with your breathing unnecessarily
- not being able to breathe deeply and fully

Consider your results and answers to the tests and questions given in this section. How do you rate your conscious breathing ability out of 10? Do you truly believe you are able to breathe to the best of your ability and that your breathing is totally versatile? Do you feel you need to improve?

Breathing in and out of the nose

The nose is intricately designed by nature for normal, everyday breathing. The nose has a sophisticated system that filters incoming air. It appropriately warms and humidifies the air, making it moist before it enters the lungs. The mucus lining leading to the lungs is sufficiently lubricated, trapping any unwanted matter, which is then swept up to the throat region, stopping it from reaching the lungs. If the air contains an irritant, like a chemical, an automatic reaction such as a sneeze, cough or shallow breath is the ideal way to breathe.

The whole system is designed to protect the lungs and prevent damage or irritation to them. Many of the airways below the nose and mouth have mucous and cilia to trap particles. However, if you breathe through your mouth, you will not be able to humidify and warm the air before it reaches the lungs. So for everyday quiet breathing, it is ideal to breathe in and out of the nose. I do not agree with breathing in with the nose and out with the mouth, or vice versa, as it breaks the rhythm and, in my opinion, seems an unnatural way to breathe. But it could be used in certain circumstances, such as during exercise or relaxation.

Many people resort to mouth breathing because they have difficulty breathing fully through their nose. For some, it may feel like a constant struggle to breathe with their nose at all, due to some structural problem with their jaw or nose. In these cases, it may be that breathing with the mouth open is a better way to breathe, as it's the only way to take a deep and satisfying breath. (You can have your mouth open and still be breathing in and out of the nose.) Furthermore, one of the most common times to breathe through the mouth is while exercising. In fact, it could be dangerous to try to breathe through the nose when exercising unless you know what you are doing or are properly trained by an expert.

However, if you don't have a problem with your everyday natural breathing that makes it difficult for you to breathe through your nose, you should be aware that continuously breathing through the mouth is one of the worst breathing habits. Remember that air, which goes through the nose, is warmed and humidified. And breathing through the mouth dries out the throat and may cause a sore throat. I strongly urge mouth breathers to do whatever it takes to get to a point where they naturally and comfortably breathe through the nose. This is simply the healthiest way to breathe. If you habitually breathe in and out of your mouth, can you pinpoint the reasons why? If you have a sinus problem, perhaps you could see someone who specializes in that field. If you have tried to breathe with your mouth closed but still find it difficult, it might be worth having your jaw and nose checked to see if there might be some structural problem.

If your nose is broken or your septum is crooked, ask advice from an ear, nose and throat specialist. As you take about 20,000 breaths everyday, it is worth the time and trouble to make sure your nasal passages are as clear as they can be.

Ideal breathing and the importance of awareness

What does it mean to be an "ideal breather," and why is it so important? Does being an expert in one type of breathing necessarily mean you automatically breathe appropriately in all circumstances? For example, one person might be an expert breather for a particular activity, such as tennis. Another person, having learned to "adapt" the breath appropriately for each different task, may use the art of breathing more effectively overall.

As previously mentioned, breathing changes constantly, according to different circumstances, and if people do not adapt their breathing successfully, they may not function to the best of their ability for a particular task. Being an expert at one type of breathing does not guarantee that you are automatically an expert in others. The breathing used for tennis is perfect for tennis. But even if someone were the best tennis player in the world, he or she would need to learn a different kind of breathing to play football, relax or sing.

For the function of resting and reading a book, passive, quiet breathing is required. It happens automatically, and you are usually not aware of your natural breathing. This kind of breathing is appropriate for the situation, and it is unnecessary to take enormous breaths to simply sit and read. However, for an activity such as running, the opposite extreme is required. What do you think would happen if you used a sitting breath for running? You do not have to be an athlete to know that you would not be able to run for very long. You need to take voluminous amounts of breath and use more lung capacity for such a strenuous activity.

An ideal breather is someone who does not resist the body's natural urge to change the breath according to the circumstances it is in. The person allows this to happen with ease, and the breath is in exact accordance with the demand.

Not appropriately adapting the breath when required is one of the main reasons for the development of impaired breathing. When our breath is inadequate—that is, when we are holding on to our breath and our breathing is not in sync with our movements—it is up to us to consciously change our breath appropriately so that our breathing is functioning harmoniously for each activity.

Imagine the following functions and think about what kind of breath is normally used: sneezing, sighing, yawning, sleeping, laughing, crying.

Now imagine the following emotional states and try to recall what kind of breathing is used: happy, ecstatic, sad, angry, guilty, nervous, frightened, shocked, irritated, shy, confident.

Next, think of the following activities and even if you have never done them, try to imagine what kind of breath would be used: walking, jogging, aerobics, running, swimming, tennis, football, basketball, cycling, weight training, bowling.

If you had to pick up two objects—one very heavy, the other very light—would you breathe exactly the same way for both or would you adjust? Naturally, you would adjust; otherwise you would not be able to pick up the heavy object. But consider exactly how you would adjust your breathing in order to pick up the heavy object. Would any kind of breathing do, or would you have to breathe a specific way?

The importance of being aware

Awareness is one of the most fundamental lessons in breathing training and without it, you will never achieve a really high quality of breathing. Most people admit to me that they have never given the "quality" of their breathing a second thought. Even if you do not ever technically learn how to improve your breathing, simply by observing how you are breathing in every circumstance you will gain certain insights that no teacher could ever give you.

EXERCISE

This is an easy exercise in awareness. All you have to do is observe how you breathe over a period of time. You don't have to do it all at once. Pick a few instances here and there throughout your day. Try it for a week or a month in order to cover a full range of situations. Initially, you might be a bit mechanical about it all. But as time goes on, you will begin to develop a sensitivity that will allow you to feel your own breathing patterns and any habits you have that interfere with your breathing. Each activity requires you to breathe in accordance with the task at hand. It is important to take note of exactly how you are breathing in everything you do. For example, how do you breathe when you are:

- at work
- waiting in traffic
- watching television
- walking casually
- walking quickly
- exercising
- cooking

- washing the car
- cleaning
- mowing the lawn

Take a moment to think about the way you breathe in each situation. Next time you actually do one of these activities, keep in mind the following questions:

- Do you feel you are breathing in the most appropriate way?
- Are you holding your breath at any point?
- Are you struggling for breath or is it adequate and in harmony with what you are doing?
- If you are struggling, can you change your breathing until you feel comfortable?
- Is your exhalation too hard? Or your inhalation too weak?
- Is your posture poor, therefore inhibiting your ability to breathe naturally or fully?

Do you relate to any of these problems? You may also want to refer back to signs of "respiratory distress," page 18.

As you become more in tune with your breathing, you will begin to be aware that many occurrences in everyday life cause changes and variations in the way you breathe. It is only when you reach this point that you are in a position to change it if you need to because you have the awareness to adjust as is necessary.

So your first task is to allow the breath to change in a way that is the most suitable for each situation. Then you will begin to see and experience how effortless tasks and activities can be. Why? Because you are breathing with your movements and not struggling against them. When you do not breathe appropriately, the same activity or situation is harder.

In the beginning, you will need to spend extra time with observation and awareness. I suggest you keep observing and experimenting until you learn how to breathe appropriately in all situations. As time passes and you become more experienced, you will know what kind of breathing is required.

When you reach this state of awareness with your breathing, it is a great sign of how far you have come. You will be able to compare your ability with a time when you had very little, if any, breathing awareness. This awareness is something you will want to maintain because of how many of us habitually hold on to our breath and/or breathe inappropriately.

I am still constantly aware of how I am breathing for certain activities. I do not see it as an effort or difficult to do, because I know by breathing ideally for each task, I will be able to perform it without unnecessary effort or struggle, and my energy will not be unnecessarily drained.

BREATHING QUIZ

Choose two different emotional states and two different activities. Make sure each pair is opposite, for example:

A) happy   B) sad
A) walking   B) running

Now write down exactly how you think you should ideally breathe in each circumstance.

Next, ask two or more people how they would breathe in the same situations. Ask as many different people as you can. The more you ask, the better the insight you will gain. Did everyone breathe the same way in the same circumstances, or were there obvious differences? How many people told you they had never thought about how they breathe—especially in different circumstances?

The breath check

What is the breath check? It is an on-going awareness exercise that can be used throughout the day, any time and anywhere, to simply keep an eye on how you are breathing in every circumstance. When you first begin breathing training, the breath check is crucial for many reasons. It allows you to realize how often you may be holding your breath. Be especially aware of whether or not you hold on to your breath in times of stress, fear, sadness, pain or exercise. If you make it a point to use the breath check to avoid inappropriately holding your breath, your overall style of breathing will dramatically improve.

THE BREATH CHECK EXERCISE

The procedure is simple. As often as possible, simply stop for a moment and bring your awareness to exactly how you are breathing. For example, when you are angry, do you tend to hold on to your breath? When you are walking up the stairs, what kind of breathing happened before, during and after? Were you breathing enough for the demand or were you breathless after only a short distance? Did you recover quickly, or were you breathless for a long time afterward?

The breath check only takes a few moments. The most important objectives of this lesson are awareness and assessment. As time goes on, you will begin to see a pattern. You will then be able to assess when you are breathing appropriately and when you are breathing inappropriately. This will begin the process of change, so that you can keep your breathing natural and undisturbed throughout the day.

The body
and
the breath

The structures involved in the act of breathing are the nose, pharynx, larynx, trachea, bronchi, lungs, diaphragm and rib cage. These structures make up the "respiratory system" and operate under various controls—mechanical, chemical and via the nervous system.

Surrounding and protecting the lungs is the thorax, made up of ribs, cartilage, breastbone and backbone. When you breathe in, oxygen enters your lungs, and the blood carries it from the lungs to all the cells of your body. Inside each cell, oxygen and glucose from food are used in a process called "respiration." Energy, carbon dioxide and water are produced during this process. Carbon dioxide is taken back to the lungs to leave the body when you breathe out. You never totally eliminate all of the carbon dioxide. And you never completely exhale all air, as there is always residual air left in the lungs.

The muscles of the chest control breathing movements. The "diaphragm" is a sheet of muscle tissue that forms the floor of your chest. The diaphragm plays the most important part in controlling the breath as it is the main muscle used for inhalation. There are other muscles between your ribs called "intercostal muscles" that can contract to move your ribs. The intercostal muscles are also involved in both inhalation and exhalation. The inspiratory intercostal muscles are not as powerful as the diaphragm. The abdominal muscles are the main muscles used for exhalation.

In respiratory physiology, we talk about two types of breathing: costal (thoracic) breathing and abdominal breathing. In abdominal breathing, lung expansion is achieved through contraction of the diaphragm. Costal breathing takes the form of shallow breathing, increasing the lung dimension through lifting up the ribs. Abdominal breathing, as opposed to costal breathing, is a more effective form of breathing.

Taking a breath into the lungs is easy enough. This occurs when the main breathing muscle, the diaphragm, along with the intercostal muscles, contract at about the same time. What follows is an expansion of the rib cage, creating suction in the lungs and consequently drawing air into the lungs.

Breathing out during quiet breathing is effortless. It is much like the emptying of a filled balloon, simply letting the air out. During active breathing, as in exercise, the thick muscles in the abdomen are recruited to expel air from the lungs. The abdominals are powerful muscles. They are needed for your daily straining during bowel motion, when you sneeze, cough, sing and during childbirth.

The type of breathing used depends on various factors such as age, the type of work or clothing worn. The aging process makes our chest wall stiffen so that we rely more on abdominal breathing. Costal breathing is naturally adopted by women during late pregnancy due to restricted abdominal breathing. Very tight clothing, such as a corset, restricts abdominal breathing. Individuals doing heavy manual work, or mountaineers, automatically assume abdominal types of breathing.

The respiratory system has been designed to take in oxygen and to eliminate carbon dioxide. If your breathing is compromised in some ways, then oxygen delivery to your cells will be harmed and the accumulation of carbon dioxide will burden your kidneys.

Everyday, we move about 8,640 liters of air in and out of the lungs, which is about 4.5 times the amount we eat or drink. A normal breath by someone who is not physically active is about 0.5 liters of air. If you are sitting all day (about eight hours), you are moving about 2,880 liters of air.

The deepest breath we can exhale after eliminating as much air as possible is about 2.5–6.5 liters, depending on age and height. When we are resting, we only use a small percentage of our total lung capacity.

BREATHING MECHANISMS

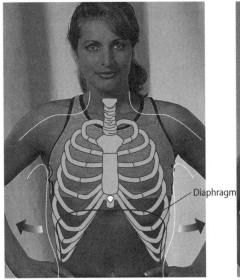
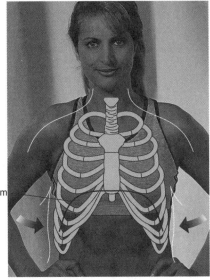

Inhalation   Exhalation

Diaphragm

The zones

There are three main areas of the body (or zones) that I refer to throughout this book: zone 1, zone 2 and zone 3.

THE ZONES

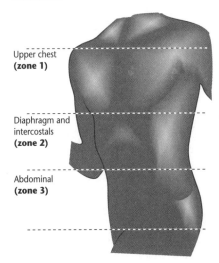

Upper chest
(zone 1)

Begins from the top of the upper lungs (just above collar bone) and finishes at the diaphragm.

Diaphragm and
intercostals
(zone 2)

Begins at the diaphragm. Place your hands on both sides of your rib cage; the width of your hand is zone 2.

Abdominal
(zone 3)

Begins where zone 2 finishes (about 3 fingers up from your belly button) and finishes at the bottom of your abdominal muscles and pelvic floor.

The type of activity you are breathing for should determine "where" you breathe to and the type of breath you use. As discussed, all parts of the respiratory system are involved at all times. However, the strength of your diaphragm, how you control it and the duration of your breath all will affect the type of breath you produce. The degree of involvement from the upper chest and the abdomen can also make a difference. For example, you will predominately use the upper chest and diaphragm during exercise, the diaphragm and abdomen for t'ai chi and martial arts, and a combination of all three for singing and yoga.

Types of breathing—physiological definitions

Before we move into the Practical training chapter of this book, it is important to clarify some physiological/technical breathing definitions.

Abdominal/diaphragmatic breathing (basic breathing)

This is the basic type of breathing.

Inspiration (inhalation)

The major muscles of inhalation are the *diaphragm* and the *external intercostal muscles.* When you breathe in, air is drawn in through your nose and/or mouth and moves down the windpipe. The windpipe divides into two bronchi, one going to the left lung and the other to the right lung. Air passes through the bronchi into a series of smaller and smaller tubes, ending in tiny air sacs called alveoli, which are surrounded by blood vessels. Oxygen from the air seeps through the walls of the alveoli into the blood. The oxygen is picked up by red blood cells and carried around the body.

Expiration (exhalation)

Expiration is normally a passive process, similar to air being released from a balloon. When an active or forceful exhalation occurs, as in exercise, it is caused by contraction of the (thick) muscles in the abdomen and the *internal intercostal muscles.*

Upper chest breathing

In upper chest breathing, the mechanics of breathing are essentially the same as described above, but there is a predominate use of the upper chest muscles to draw in and expel the breath. Upper chest breathing brings in a smaller volume of air compared with abdominal/diaphragmatic breathing.

Types of breathing—practical definitions

First of all I want to explain why I divide the breath into three types of breathing when in basic physiology, there are only two types of breathing: upper chest and abdominal/diaphragmatic.

I deliberately divide the second category in two in order to teach different styles of breathing more effectively. Therefore, the three main types of breathing referred to in this book are upper chest breathing, diaphragmatic breathing, and abdominal breathing. Other breathing terms are used to illustrate and instruct these breathing styles.

If you have knowledge in respiratory physiology, you may be thinking at this point that the diaphragm is always used for respiration with abdominal movement, so why create three categories?

I created separate definitions because of the feedback I have received over the years—particularly from proficient abdominal breathers—as well as my own experience from practicing with the breath. I achieve different results when the diaphragm and/or lower ribs are the focus of movement, compared with when the focus is on the abdomen.

People think of me as a "breathing coach" similar to that of a singing teacher. My role as a breathing coach is to help people in a practical sense. People who come to me do so in order to enhance their breathing for a particular purpose. Most of them know nothing about physiology; they simply want to improve their breathing.

The way I help them to achieve this is by using my own specific terms and visual images, as well as personally demonstrating breathing techniques. The important aim for me is that average individuals can relate to my way of teaching and achieve positive changes with their breathing as a result.

The following definitions give you an overview of the terminology I refer to during breathing training. Some of the terms will be described in more detail later in the book.

Breathing training

This basically means to improve and develop your breathing. We all need to do some form of breathing training for our general health. Some will also choose certain forms of breathing training for their specific needs. Breathing training covers two kinds: "external" and "Internal."

External breathing training

Everyone is familiar with external breathing training. It is breathing that happens automatically as a result of exercise or any demanding bodily movement.

Internal breathing training

This is a manner of deep breathing that happens by your conscious effort. There is either no bodily movement, and you are lying or sitting still, or there is movement that is usually slow and gentle. Internal breathing can still occur with fast movement, but the emphasis on "how" you breathe is different when compared with general exercise. With demanding movements, a combination of internal and external breathing occurs. Specifically how you breathe during demanding movements can determine whether it is predominately internal or external breathing that is occurring.

Internal and external breathing will be covered in greater detail on pages 120–122.

Terminology for ways you can breathe

Nose/mouth breathing—"strong" and "passive"

It is possible to breathe in and out of the nose with your mouth open, but this manner of breathing refers to inhaling and exhaling through the mouth. There are times when mouth breathing can be a more effective way of breathing, for example during exercise. Particularly for unfit people, this method of breathing is essential for any kind of strenuous or demanding activity.

There are varying degrees of mouth breathing. On a scale of 1 to 10, with 1 being gentle and 10 being powerful, you could use a level of 2 for relaxation and an 8 when you are jogging up a steep hill. You need to experiment. Learn how to breathe in and out of the mouth in a soft and gentle manner and just as proficiently in a strong and dynamic way.

Sniff breathing and throat breathing

"Throat" and "sniff breathing" are two terms that I have created and commonly use whenever I am teaching breathing. Obviously, the nose or throat itself doesn't breathe, so technically, there is no such concept. In my teaching, these terms help to describe different styles of breathing and the sensations that are predominately felt in particular areas when using these kinds of breath. The difference between the two is that the focus of attention is in the throat area for throat breathing and the nasal area for sniff breathing. But the basic mechanics of breathing, physiologically speaking, are the same for both of them. So "sniff" and "throat breathing" are kinesthetic (sensations) terms, not physiological ones.

Sniff breathing

This is how I describe a shallow, upper chest breath. With this kind of breathing, the sensation of airflow is predominately felt in the nasal area. It involves a short and sharp intake of breath, exactly like a sniff, with the upper chest lifting as well. The exhalation is also expelled quickly with the upper chest dropping.

This style of breathing can't be properly regulated and controlled. Sniff breathing results in drawing in too much breath too soon and exhaling too much air too rapidly. If you continue to try to draw in a longer breath in this manner, you will find that you struggle with your breathing and automatically tighten up. This tension instantly cuts the breath short in an abrupt manner. This kind of breathing consequently produces a weak and poor quality breath. Doing too much of it continuously can make you feel light-headed or dizzy.

Throat breathing

Throat breathing is the term used to describe the sensation that is felt with the muscles in the throat when breathing deeply. Whether breathing occurs through the nose or mouth, the focus is still perceived in the throat area. Throat breathing is the kind of breathing that happens naturally when good quality deep breathing occurs. By consciously learning how to throat breathe, you can control and regulate the breath. You will also be able to produce different kinds of breathing, thereby giving you great versatility. Instructions on page 53 will teach you how to use throat breathing to take the breath deeper, softer, stronger, longer, shorter, and to vary the intensity of a breath.

The sound also gives you the opportunity to monitor and observe the quality and duration of your breathing. When throat breathing is performed properly, a feeling of calmness and relaxation is typically felt by all who experience it. The smooth and gentle rhythmic breathing helps the body to relax muscular tension. And the sound produced is calming; it helps to soothe the mind, especially when people feel stressed.

Shallow breathing

Shallow upper chest breathing

With this kind of breathing, air is pulled in mainly to the upper region of the lungs. Once the air is drawn in, it is very quickly exhaled. The breath can also be erratic at times. In this manner, only a small portion of the entire lung capacity is used, with less air reaching the lower part of the lungs. When shallow breathing persists, it can lead to many mental and physical problems, including anxiety and stress.

**INCORRECT
INHALATION**

**INCORRECT
EXHALATION**

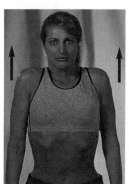

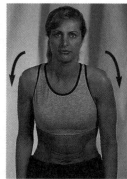

Here is a front view of a shallow breath in its exaggerated form. It is a quick, short breath predominately pulled in by the muscles of the chest, which mainly reach the upper part of the lungs. When exhaling, the chest and shoulders drop downward.

Shoulders and upper chest are lifted.

Shoulders and upper chest have dropped downward. The whole posture is out of alignment.

**CORRECT
INHALATION**

**CORRECT
EXHALATION**

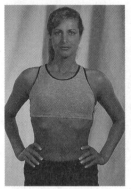

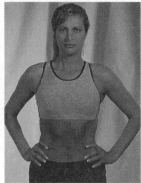

For good quality breathing to occur, the upper chest should stay this way for the inhalation and the exhalation.

Chin is comfortably toward the chest, torso is lengthened, shoulders and chest are upright and opened, and the neck is lengthened.

Posture stays the same as for the inhalation.

When breathing naturally, and if you are training to achieve good quality breathing, shallow upper chest breathing is discouraged. The main reason is because it can become habitual, and eventually detrimental to one's health both physically and mentally. During exercise in particular, continuous upper chest breathing without major involvement of the diaphragm, and the (thick) abdominal muscles, can have a tiring effect, as most unfit people often experience.

However, there are times when upper chest breathing is needed. For example, in a dangerous situation, upper chest breathing is often a natural and necessary reaction. In my opinion, upper chest breathing can be used in a positive way. It is actually incorporated as part of a complete yoga breath. And the fit athlete you admire is using upper chest breathing. But, they are also maximizing the use of their diaphragms and abdominal muscles in every way possible. So to clarify, I do not recommend the habitual and continual use of "shallow" upper chest breathing. Otherwise, upper chest breathing can be properly incorporated at appropriate times as part of a breathing style when it also includes a predominate use of the diaphragm.

Stressful breathing

Shallow and erratic breathing, which does not have a harmonious rhythm, are characteristics of stressful breathing. It typically occurs during a stressful situation and can produce a feeling of lethargy and increased tension in the body. Intermittently holding your breath in stressful moments can contribute to stressful breathing, as can continual sniff breathing, as described previously (see page 32).

Deep breathing

The following are definitions of all kinds of deep breathing. I will expand some of them further in the next section. They all produce a good quality deep breath when performed properly.

Abdominal/diaphragmatic breathing

Deep breathing is a good quality breath that is basically an extended version of the abdominal/diaphragmatic breath explained on page 30. All abdominal/diaphragmatic breathing uses throat breathing. The diaphragm and abdominal muscles are the muscles predominately used, with no unnecessary or exaggerated movement from the upper chest and shoulders. The characteristics of relaxed deep breathing are rhythmical, elongated and slow breaths. This is the kind of breathing that naturally occurs when you are in a deep sleep or feeling relaxed. However, deep breathing can also be strong and powerful.

Abdominal breathing

Abdominal breathing is the most universally known and used method of deep breathing. In breathing training, abdominal breathing is commonly regarded as the easiest and yet extremely effective style of breathing for the relaxation of the mind and body. The emphasis is on the abdomen being the focal point with an obvious movement on both the inhalation and the exhalation and no exaggerated movement from the upper chest area.

The abdomen elevates and expands on the inhalation and depresses and decreases in size on the exhalation as a result of the diaphragm moving downward and upward respectively. A deep inhalation involved in an abdominal breath allows the abdomen to be fully pushed forward; then returns to the original position on the exhalation. (The best analogy is to think of air moving in and out of a balloon.)

Relaxation breathing

Abdominal breathing, which is long, slow, deep and even, is classified as relaxation breathing. This whole manner of breathing is conducive to resting and mentally and physically unwinding. Once mastered and performed properly, relaxation breathing can result in a very deep state of relaxation.

Yoga breathing

The complete yoga breath is divided into three parts using all three zones of the body: 1. clavicular (upper), 2. intercostal (middle), and 3. abdominal (lower). Before combining all three parts, it is standard practice to learn the three separately. They are combined to achieve one continual, harmonious and rhythmical movement—similar to a wave. It is one of the best methods of breathing to produce a relaxed mind and body.

So how does yoga breathing differ from other forms of breathing training? I have put this question to a number of yoga practitioners. The common answer is that yoga breathing has a very sedating and calming effect on the mind and body. Thousands of people around the world would testify to the incredible benefits of yoga breathing for physical and mental relaxation.

THE YOGA INHALATION

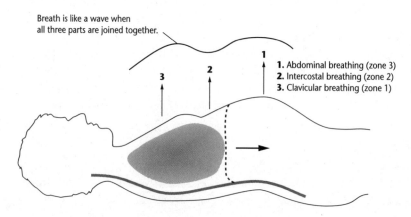

Breath is like a wave when all three parts are joined together.

1. Abdominal breathing (zone 3)
2. Intercostal breathing (zone 2)
3. Clavicular breathing (zone 1)

THE YOGA EXHALATION

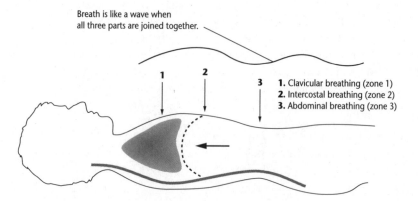

Breath is like a wave when all three parts are joined together.

1. Clavicular breathing (zone 1)
2. Intercostal breathing (zone 2)
3. Abdominal breathing (zone 3)

What is the diaphragm?

Unless you have a physiology background, you probably have no idea what the diaphragm actually is or how to control it. Yet the diaphragm plays a major role in drawing in air, which therefore makes it one of the most important muscles in keeping us alive. It is a thin muscle lying horizontally separating the lungs from the abdomen (see page 29). It is one of the hardest working muscles of the body, and like any muscle, it can be trained so that it is strengthened and relaxed. You can consciously control your diaphragm and command it to do different tasks. Opera singers in particular are very aware of the diaphragm and how it can be strengthened and controlled in order to adapt the breath to suit whatever note they are singing.

Diaphragmatic breathing

Diaphragmatic breathing, as opposed to abdominal breathing, is not typically known about, however it is one of the most powerful and effective methods of good quality breathing. This is a much more challenging method of breathing to learn compared with abdominal breathing. The focal points and emphasis are the diaphragm, lower rib cage and abdomen. The diaphragm is the strongest muscle for breathing, especially for inhalation. This method of breathing involves the predominate use of the diaphragm assisted by the intercostal muscles and abdominal muscles. There is an obvious and powerful movement of the rib cage inward and outward (similar to bellows). There is no obvious movement from the upper chest and shoulders and minimal movement from the abdomen.

One of the reasons athletes and singers can control their breathing is that they *all* have a strong and toned diaphragm. By controlling the diaphragm in specific ways, you can determine the "kind" of breath you produce, and therefore adjust it according to the demand. To produce different kinds of good quality breathing, using the relevant breathing muscles makes a big difference. In particular, your specific application of throat breathing and the diaphragm are the two most important aspects to achieve successful results. Only when the diaphragm is fully involved can you breathe the most efficiently and meet the demands of a strenuous activity.

An effective way to strengthen the diaphragm is to learn to vigorously move it without an exaggerated use of zone 1 and as little of zone 3 as possible. By doing this, you can totally control the diaphragm and dynamically move the rib cage to accommodate even the most demanding activities. This gives you excellent control and can create a much more powerful movement than merely lifting and dropping your rib cage with your shoulders and upper chest.

Power breathing

Power breathing is the most dynamic method of breathing. It is employed in all power sports, for example when sprinting or lifting heavy weights. The diaphragm is used to its maximum potential, and the rib cage moves inward and outward in short, vigorous bursts to create deep, powerful breaths. You will have a feeling of energy and vitality once power breathing has been mastered. It is an extremely effective way of strengthening the diaphragm, lungs and the overall breathing apparatus.

What is the difference between diaphragmatic and abdominal breathing?

ABDOMINAL INHALATION   **ABDOMINAL EXHALATION**

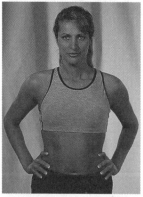 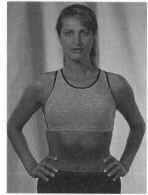

The emphasis is on moving the abdomen.

DIAPHRAGMATIC INHALATION   **DIAPHRAGMATIC EXHALATION**

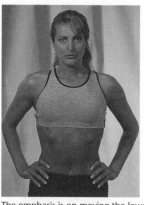 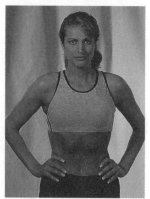

The emphasis is on moving the lower rib cage.

The diaphragm and abdomen function very closely together during the act of breathing. But I believe it is important to learn them as separate types of breathing in order to be more versatile with your breathing (see pages 30–31).

Certainly, everyone should learn abdominal breathing, but it is also important to become proficient in diaphragmatic breathing. Diaphragmatic breathing helps you to significantly strengthen your diaphragm, which gives you more control over your breathing and you can adapt it to suit different circumstances and activities, whereas abdominal breathing is the better choice for relaxation.

The specific breathing drills that are a part of diaphragmatic breathing training in this book will help you to strengthen the diaphragm much more effectively than basic abdominal breathing. Also, while abdominal breathing does expand the ribs more than a standard breath does, it is only by working the diaphragm in a specific way that you create a really dynamic and powerful movement with the ribs, which is achieved by diaphragmatic breathing.

People who are experienced at abdominal breathing come to me in order to explore another angle of breathing. Even teachers and experts in singing, diving, martial arts, yoga and t'ai chi are amazed at the difference they experience after learning how to further control and strengthen the diaphragm. Many of them are able to take up new activities they previously struggled with or simply could not do, such as running or swimming.

These specialists ask me why there is such a difference with their breathing when they already knew how to breathe well. My answer is that although they are highly adept with abdominal breathing, or whatever specialized breathing they use for their particular activity, it is still only one type of breathing. I teach a variety of different breathing techniques aimed at strengthening and coordinating all aspects of the breathing apparatus.

Picture a t'ai chi master and a world-class sprinter. In t'ai chi, breathing is used to bring energy to the power center, which is termed "Dan Tian." It is a grounding breath that t'ai chi masters believe keeps you centered, stores energy and builds great internal power. It is typically a long, slow, deep and even breath. The sprinter, on the other hand, needs a powerful, explosive, quick moving breath. The t'ai chi method of breathing could not be used by someone wanting to run fast, and the breathing method required for running is totally inappropriate for t'ai chi. They are two diverse methods of breathing.

For both types of breathing, however, the diaphragm is the most important muscle. The t'ai chi master could develop his breathing from another angle (externally) if he were to run fast, and the runner could also enhance his breathing (internally) by doing t'ai chi. A singer, athlete or anyone else can effectively improve breathing by challenging it differently from what they are used to.

The following comments are from some of my clients after they have learned diaphragmatic breathing:

I feel I have maximum control with my whole manner of breathing and can create any kind of breath I want for any particular purpose.

There is a significant increase in how long I can breathe in and out, which therefore means I increase how much I fill up my lung capacity.

My abdominal breathing greatly improved as a result of my diaphragm becoming toned and stronger.

I can move my rib cage inward and outward (like an accordion) creating a very powerful movement. I can fully control my diaphragm and now I have an increased ability to effectively change my style of breathing for numerous activities.

Breathing patterns

We can clearly see how all kinds of breathing have some similar qualities that overlap one another. For example, abdominal and yoga breathing both have a calming effect. But each style of breathing has one or more distinct qualities that make it the ideal breathing technique to use for that particular circumstance.

According to the feedback I was constantly receiving, there seemed to be a correlation between certain breathing patterns and how a person feels or acts. I became intrigued when I observed that when people breathed a certain way, they felt a similar feeling, both physically and mentally. Different breaths produced distinctly different effects.

Years later, I was fascinated to learn from physiologists that on special machines used to record different types of breathing, erratic breathing recorded differently than deep breathing. I was given the opportunity to personally test different breathing techniques on a couple of different machines and with different people who were experts in this field. I found that there was a definite and obvious difference recorded between breathing patterns. Each breathing technique produced its own kind of result. This helped explain my personal experience as well as confirming what numerous people have reported to me over the years.

So based on my own and my clients' experiences, I concluded that how you breathe, whether it is shallow or deep, quick or slow, can influence and affect how you feel and perform physically. Think of these two examples: a long, slow and deep breath makes a person feel relaxed. On the other hand, a sharp burst of breath, as in the case of lifting a heavy weight, gives a feeling of explosive energy and alertness. If you deliberately tried to do the opposite breaths for either task, do you think you could perform equally as well or achieve the same results?

All you need to understand is that certain kinds of breathing produce particular breathing patterns, which produce different effects. It is a matter of finding out what is the best way of breathing for the task at hand. Experiment for yourself to see what physical and mental effect each kind of breathing has on you.

The two graphs below demonstrate test results from the University of Sydney for experiments conducted by Dr. Chin Moi Chow. These show the difference between deep and erratic breathing.

DEEP BREATHING

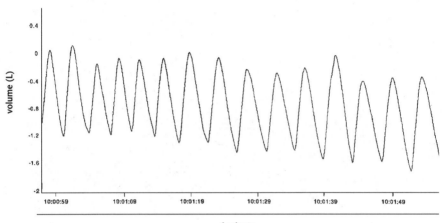

1 minute

ERRATIC BREATHING

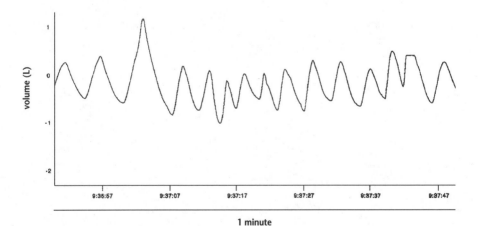

1 minute

PRACTICAL TRAINING

Getting ready for breathing training

You should be aware of a few important facts before we commence the practical training.

Using sound for feedback

You must pay particular attention to the sound of your breath during breathing training because it will give you a good indication of exactly what is going on. Sound can tell you about:

- the quality, depth and power of the breath
- what kind of breath is happening at any particular moment
- the consistency
- the exact duration
- how much control you have

When it comes to good quality breathing, there is a particular sound that must be produced, which happens as a result of breathing deeply. You will experience this when you practice throat breathing. It is the first crucial step in learning good quality breathing, which will be covered in more detail later.

Balancing the breath

When consciously improving the quality of your breathing, it is very important to breathe in and out equally, in strength and duration. Many of you will find that it is easier to keep improving the exhalation, but in this way the inhalation can be, and often is, neglected. To develop only half of the breath creates an imbalance. Most forms of breathing training concentrate on increasing the quality and duration of the exhalation, to the detriment of the inhalation.

Why this is so, I do not know as I believe each is as important as the other. I can only guess that it is assumed the inhalation will automatically be as good as the exhalation (not true, according to my test results on clients). Also, for most tasks, the emphasis is on the exhalation.

In regard to achieving high standards in breathing training, it is crucial that you develop your inhalation and control it like you can your exhalation. Even though your exhalation will more than likely always be better than your inhalation, you should still aim to keep them reasonably even in quality and duration (i.e., your inhalation should be as long and as strong as your exhalation). When developing the breath, it is very important to try to bring the standard of the inhalation and the exhalation to the same point, rather than have them obviously unbalanced—for example, when trying to breathe deeply, continuously pushing out too hard on the exhalation and pulling in far less breath weakly on the inhalation.

Why is the exhalation stronger than the inhalation?

During normal quiet breathing, expiration is an entirely passive process, without active use of any muscles. But in many situations, such as during exercise or singing, exhalations need to be forceful. Our bodies are designed so that there are powerful muscles to expel air—such as during a sneeze or a cough to eject a dangerous object caught in the throat. Instinct tells us to blow out candles on a cake, not breathe in. In order to speak or sing, we must breathe out. The ability to exhale forcibly is innate, so it is obvious why the exhalation is stronger and more developed than the inhalation in these circumstances.

However, when learning different methods of breathing, for example relaxation breathing, I have found a common problem is to *unnecessarily* push out too hard on the exhalation. And in most instances, the inhalation is much shorter and weaker, with an inability to make it longer and stronger if needed. But this does not mean we cannot develop a strong inhalation. In actual fact, we have the ability for our inhalation to also be powerful and strong. We can also learn how to soften and lengthen the exhalation.

Balancing the breath is an area usually neglected, but it is something I feel is of the utmost importance. Some of the singers I have worked with, as well as others with well-developed exhalations, tell me they noticed a marked improvement once they fully developed their inhalation as well.

If like most people, you find it easier to develop the exhalation, spend extra time on developing your inhalation until it is as good, or at least almost as good. This means working on strengthening and prolonging the inhalation. No matter how much extra work you need to do initially to balance your breathing, you will notice a significant improvement in time.

Lengthening and softening the breath

The first important task in building the foundation for quality breathing is to learn how to breathe more slowly, gently, longer and deeply. While there are numerous variations in breathing, all of them come after this basic training. When you have this foundation in place, all that will follow will fall into place naturally.

In building this foundation, you will learn how to effectively regulate the flow of your breath, enabling you to continuously lengthen your breath for the inhalation and exhalation. Once you master this, you will see how easy it is to control your breathing in any way that suits your needs, including strengthening the breath for power breathing. And importantly, you will be able to adjust your breathing to suit any demand, therefore making you an adaptable and versatile breather.

When people start breathing training and I ask them to show me their best quality breath, one of the biggest and most common problems I see is an abrupt breath, like a gasp, with an inability to breathe in or out for more than a few seconds.

Why should you learn to lengthen your breath?

- Lengthened breathing is the foundation upon which all good quality breathing is based.

- It induces relaxation in the mind and body.

- The diaphragm needs to be relaxed and strengthened, as do all muscles. By practicing lengthened breathing, the flexibility of your breathing apparatus will be increased.

Why should you learn to strengthen your breathing?

Most people find it difficult to strengthen their breathing, especially on the inhalation. It is very rare to find someone who inhales too powerfully, who needs to learn to soften it. The ideal is to be able to breathe as softly and gently as possible, but also as strongly and as powerfully as possible. It is common for most people to find it more difficult to strengthen the inhalation—but that is usually because the correct technique is not applied.

Strengthening the breath is required because there are times when you need to pull in or expel a powerful breath. Also, power breathing is one of the best ways to tone up your breathing muscles, especially the diaphragm. Breathing powerfully gives you incredible versatility. Being able only to breathe softly would limit your full range of potential, as there are times that only a strong and powerful breath will be able to meet the need. So your task is to learn how to breathe strongly and powerfully for a few seconds and also for a slightly extended period of time. While this is one of the most difficult parts of breathing training, it will bring rewards. When performing demanding tasks that require strength and power, you will feel strong, energized, refreshed and alert!

Timing the breath

It's important to assess your breathing *before* you begin breathing training, so you can use it as a measure for your progress. Timing how long you can breathe is not the only factor to consider; the quality of breath is more important. However, timing is simply a gauge for you to note how your duration improves as you practice, which then reflects the quality and your ability to control your breath.

First of all, you will need a stopwatch preferably or a watch or a clock with a second hand. We are going to do four timings:

- inhalation using the nose only
- exhalation using the nose only
- inhalation using the mouth only
- exhalation using the mouth only

While nose breathing is best for everyday breathing, I suggest that you also time how long you can breathe in and out of your mouth, particularly if you are interested in developing your breath for exercise and sports.

When adults consciously attempt to take their longest and deepest breath, I have found the average duration for most people's inhalation is two to four seconds and the average exhalation is four to six seconds. If you are experienced in some form of breathing training your timing may be higher, at least for the exhalation. I have found that when most people time themselves, or others, they usually overestimate. When I time them, they are almost always in the average range I have mentioned. So try to be as precise as you can, making sure you listen very carefully to the breath. You could also ask someone else to listen to your breath and time you for accuracy.

EXERCISE

The most accurate way to time yourself is by counting your breath according to sound, not bodily movement. You do not have to be breathing in order to move your shoulders or drop your chest. So count only to the last second that you can hear the breath, irrespective of whether any body parts are still moving.

Prepare yourself to time your longest breath. Make sure your mouth is completely closed and breathe in for as long as you possibly can. Then do the same for your exhalation. You will probably find that your exhalation is longer. This is normal.

NOSE

DATE							
INHALATION							
EXHALATION							

MOUTH

DATE							
INHALATION							
EXHALATION							

Creating the right environment for breathing training

Where?

Especially in the initial stages, a noisy environment is not conducive to learning how to breathe deeply and in a relaxed manner. You need a quiet environment where you can clearly hear yourself breathe. Make sure the room is at a suitable temperature. Do not expose yourself to a draft or allow yourself to get cold, as it will interfere with relaxed breathing.

When?

When you first begin learning basic breathing lessons, you will need to pick a time when you are feeling reasonably relaxed and not too stressed. Don't rush through the instructions too quickly, especially if you have not had previous breathing training. Patience will be required until you have learned the basics well. For example, if you do not learn how to throat breathe properly, then the rest of the training will not be as effective. So be prepared to stay at each particular stage until you have grasped it, before you move on.

How?

The sequence in which the breathing instructions are presented is important. I have put everything in a particular order so that you can build a foundation and progress as and when you are ready. After you have completed the preliminary exercises, and the basic breathing training, you may then go back and spend more time on any aspect you want to develop. In fact, I encourage that.

I strongly suggest that, once you have been through the entire training program, you assess yourself again and determine your weaker points. Most people find that one of their major weaknesses is the inhalation. After spending extra time working on the inhalation itself, it would be a good idea to then go back and do the whole basic session again, i.e., the inhalation and exhalation together.

Anything else I should be aware of?

I have never had any negative feedback from anybody practicing the breathing at home. Under my personal instruction, no one has experienced any difficulty. But as most of you will be working without supervision, I want to bring a few possible problems to your attention because you will not have anyone to monitor you.

If you do become dizzy, feel faint, hyperventilate (or anything else that does not feel right), then immediately stop whatever it is that you are doing until you feel you have recuperated. If you have not recovered after a short while and you keep experiencing these symptoms, stop for a couple of hours or wait until the next day.

Those problems occur because of an imbalance of carbon dioxide and oxygen. It is usually a result of pushing out too hard on the exhalation and forcibly gasping for the inhalation, so you should soften your exhalation and gently lengthen your inhalation more. Aim to keep the breath equal rather than exhaling more than you inhale. Also, proceed more slowly with the training procedure. Allow more recovery time, and limit the length of time you work. As you become used to deeper breathing, and as your breathing improves and becomes more balanced, you will be able to breathe voluminous amounts of air and feel perfectly fine.

Where do we start?

First we start by "unlearning." You cannot force your breathing to change no matter how hard you try. The most effective way is to release the blocks that are interfering with your natural breathing. If you are straining, you will not get very far in improving the quality or depth of your breathing. So if you feel any kind of tension or discomfort at any time, it is because you are inappropriately tensing the muscles (unconsciously and out of habit), constricting the flow of relaxed breathing.

The very first task is to make sure you are allowing the breath to move freely on its own. It must be neither too hard nor too weak. This is crucial and is the foundation for any breathing training. After a period of time, you may experience a sensation with your breathing that seems strange. You may feel you are breathing much better than you used to, that your whole manner of breathing is effortless and performed with ease. This is the result of no longer struggling and straining with your breath. It is a breakthrough point because it is a sign that you have eliminated improper breathing habits. It means you have loosened up and released the locked-in tightness in the muscles that interfered with your ability to breathe deeply.

Using affirmations

In breathing training, only breathing slowly and with control can lay the foundation for learning how to breathe deeply. The first three seconds of inhaling or exhaling can determine what kind of breath you will have. When aiming to breathe as deeply as possible, repeating the following phrases during those first seconds can be helpful as you consciously try to slow down and lengthen your breathing.

I've got all the time in the world to breathe. (Before you start.)

I've got all the time in the world to breathe in. (While inhaling.)

I've got all the time in the world to breathe out. (While exhaling.)

If you find yourself rushing and find it difficult to slow down, try thinking these thoughts, particularly before you start and especially for the first three seconds:

I am going to breathe in as s-l-o-w-l-y as I possibly can. (inhalation)

Or,

I am going to breathe out as s-l-o-w-l-y as I possibly can. (exhalation)

It is crucial to understand that for lengthened breathing, you must not breathe in or out as much as you can in the first few seconds. You need to breathe in or out a little bit at a time over as long a period as possible. Try to think of your breath as broken up into small components so that you can lengthen it. One of the most helpful thoughts to tell yourself is:

My breathing is made up of small components.

Other helpful thoughts are:

I am going to breathe in/out in a calm, smooth manner.

I am going to lengthen each breath for as long as I comfortably can.

I am in total control of the way I breathe in and out.

I have the ability to control how to breathe as I choose.

I choose to breathe in/out calmly and slowly.

The breath assessment questionnaire

Your next task is to do a visual breath assessment. In front of a mirror, with a bare chest or a sports top, take the biggest, longest and best quality breath that you can possibly take. Repeat this breath a few times to get an idea of how you breathe and repeat it as many times as you like throughout the questionnaire.

Did you breathe in through your nose or mouth? _____

Did you breathe out through your nose or mouth? _____

If you answer "mouth" to either, is this how you normally breathe throughout the day or only when you take a deep breath? _____

For the rest of the assessment, breathe in with your nose only. Keep your mouth completely closed.

We will first assess the inhalation. Draw your best breath in through your nose only for as long as you can.

Did the upper chest move at all? _____

If so, was it predominately or only a little? _____

Did your chest feel like it tightened up while you breathed in? _____

Did you lift your shoulders up as you breathed in? _____

Did your whole torso seem to lift as well? _____

Did your abdominal area expand? _____

Did both your abdominal and chest area expand? If so, one at a time, or both together? _____

Inhaling again, observe the *quality* and *sound* of the breath.

Was your inhalation short, erratic, fragile? _____

Was your inhalation strong and powerful or soft or weak? _____

Did you breathe in with what seemed like great urgency or did you take your time? _____

Did you gasp or struggle to breathe in or was it easy? _____

Did you feel like you could have breathed in more but somehow felt stuck at a certain point? _____

How did it sound: quiet, weak, soft, smooth, erratic, strong, powerful or anything else? _____

We will repeat the same procedure for the exhalation.

Breathe out of your nose (with your mouth closed) aiming for the best quality exhalation you can manage for as long as you can.

Did your upper chest drop as you breathed out? _____

If so, was it from the start, middle or end of the breath? _____

Did your chest drop a lot or only a little? _____

Did your abdominal area move inward or outward? _____

Did you move only the abdominal area or was it with the upper chest as well? _____

If so, which part moved first? _____

Which part moved the most? _____

Did you hunch over and roll your shoulders forward? If so, from the start, middle or end? _____

Once again, breathing out your best and longest breath through your nose only, carefully observe the quality and sound.

Was your exhale short, erratic, fragile?_____

Was your exhale strong and powerful, or soft and weak? _____

Did you expel the breath with what seemed like great urgency or did you take your time? _____

Did you struggle and force the breath out or was it easy?_____

Do you feel like you could have breathed out more but somehow felt unable to continue? _____

How did it sound: quiet, weak, soft, smooth, erratic, strong, powerful or anything else? _____

We will now assess both the inhalation and the exhalation as one. With your mouth closed, breathe in and out of your nose a few times. Once again, make it your best quality breath and for as long as you possibly can.

Which part/s moves the most: upper chest, shoulders, rib cage, abdomen? _____

What part/s moves first? _____

What part/s moves last? _____

Is there a big difference in duration between your inhalation and exhalation? If so, which is shorter? _____

Is there a big difference in quality between the two?_____

Which breath sounds weaker? _____

Which do you feel more comfortable with and why? _____

_____

After doing this assessment, take a moment to think of what you felt and observed. Now reflect on the times in your life that your breathing stopped you from participating in certain activities that you really wanted to do. _____

_____

_____

Write down what you feel are your particular problems. It could be that your chest tightens up very easily, or that you do not have flexibility around the rib cage area, or that when you get stressed, your breathing is greatly affected. _____

_____

_____

Write the main reasons why you want to improve your breathing, and the goals you would like to achieve by learning different breathing techniques._____

_____

_____

Throat breathing

In yoga, throat breathing is referred to as "ujaii breathing" and in karate, it is called "ibuki breathing." Throat breathing is linked to deep breathing because it is the way you automatically breathe when you predominately work your diaphragm, which is distinctly different from the kind of breath that happens when you are shallow breathing.

Throat breathing serves as a basis for being able to control and regulate both your inhalation and your exhalation. When I am teaching someone how to breathe a good quality breath, the first concept I teach is how to throat breathe, and I do not continue with the rest of the training until they have grasped it. Once you learn how to throat breathe properly, you have laid the initial foundation. You will then find it easier to learn how to control not only the depth of your breath, but also the relevant body parts involved.

Everybody has the ability to throat breathe because it is basically a method of deep breathing that the body innately knows how to do and often does. At some time or other, we all breathe deeply whether it is while we are sleeping or when we are in a relaxed state. So when we learn the technique of throat breathing, we are actually becoming aware of something we already know how to do; therefore, it is simply a matter of learning how to do it consciously.

SNIFF BREATHING EXERCISE

In order to identify exactly what throat breathing "isn't," let's try some sniff breathing. Imagine if you had to sniff something really hard. Now take a couple of quick breaths into and out of your upper chest, using the muscles of your nose like a suction pump. The duration should only be a few seconds for the inhalation and about the same for the exhalation. If you become dizzy, then immediately stop—you have performed it correctly!

For deep breathing, it is necessary to change your emphasis and awareness to the muscles in the throat area. When we throat breathe, we can breathe in and out of either the nose or the mouth. It is best to try throat breathing on the exhalation with the mouth first, because it is easier to grasp.

THROAT BREATHING EXERCISE

First, become aware of the appropriate muscles by clearing your throat or gently coughing. When you do this, take note of which muscles are used in the throat area, because they are the exact same muscles that will be emphasized any time you need to do throat breathing.

Make sure that your face and body are relaxed, especially the upper chest area. Now, say the word "HA" so it sounds like a sigh. Next, keep extending the "H" like this:

HHHHHHHHHHHHHHHHHHHHHHHHHHHHHHHHHHH

Extend the "H" continuously so it sounds like a gentle wind. You will find that you need to grip the back of the throat muscles to make the sound. As you make the sound, mentally and physically be aware of exactly what is happening in the throat area. If you force the exhalation too much, you will cut the breath short, so it is important for both the throat and breath to be relaxed. Be aware that there is no need to release all the breath at once. So take your time. Make sure your mind and body are relaxed, particularly your face and upper chest area. Tell yourself: "I've got all the time in the world to breathe out."

This thought will take away the urgency. Simply relax, and take all the time you need to lengthen and smooth out the exhalation as much as possible.

You will know you are throat breathing if you can breathe out for much longer than you could when you did the sniff breath. You will also notice the difference in the sound between the two. You will sense the noise emanating from the nasal area in sniff breathing, and it is forceful and quick. The sound is smoother, creating a calming sensation, when it comes from the back of the throat as it does in throat breathing.

Only when you have managed the throat breath properly on the exhalation should you attempt it on the inhalation. Initially, most people find the inhalation much harder to grasp, so don't despair or give up! Use the sound of the exhalation to give you an idea of what is needed to be achieved for the inhalation. You will still be making the continuous "H" sound, but in reverse.

Take a moment to remind yourself: "I've got all the time in the world to breathe in." Relax your mind and body. Then place your fingers on your belly button. With your mouth open, imagine drawing the breath into the belly button area, and moving the belly button outward, away from your spine as you are inhaling. Try it now until you feel comfortable with it. Aim to continuously inhale as slowly and softly and for as long as possible. Once you have achieved it with the mouth closed, perform an exhalation, using the throat muscles with a slightly stronger force and begin to really expel the air. Try it with your mouth open first, until you feel the sensation of airflow in the throat area. Then try it with the mouth closed so you are only breathing through your nose. If you still feel you are not able to throat breathe at all, then just keep trying. Everybody who has attempted it with me has been able to do it. Just accept the fact that you already know how to do throat breathing. It is a matter of your approaching it confidently, knowing the ability is already there, and learning this way of breathing consciously.

A helpful method for the inhalation is to closely observe what you did on the exhalation and simply reverse the process. Persevere until the sound and sensation you experienced during the exhalation has also been achieved for the inhalation. Try to breathe in 10 times more slowly and softly to remove that feeling of urgency. Totally relax your face and upper chest muscles as you breathe in. Keep reminding yourself: "I've got all the time in the world to breathe in." The more relaxed you are and the less you struggle, the easier you will find it to draw in the breath smoothly and for an extended period of time.

Go through the whole procedure again. Clear your throat and be aware of the muscles being used. Extend the "H" on "HA." If you feel you are unable to grasp it now, take a break, and check if you have any of the following problems. Are you tightening the head, neck and shoulders? Pulling in too much breath? Breathing in too quickly? Breathing in too hard?

The breath stops immediately if it is pulled in too abruptly. So really soften the breath, take your time, and aim to continuously pull the breath in as gently as possible, otherwise you will not achieve the desired results.

After you have achieved a basic standard with your ability to throat breathe, it is very important that you learn to fine-tune it. It is like being able to change a thermostat or the gears to your car. There are times when you need to be able to breathe long and softly; at other times, short and softly; or short, dynamic and powerful; long, strong and powerful; or of medium intensity (i.e., in between hard and soft for both a long and short breath).

You cannot apply only one standard throat breath to your breathing requirements, and there are many kinds to choose from for specific activities (all deep breathing uses throat breathing. The relaxation breath works best with a long, smooth and gentle breath. The power breath is not the power breath unless you are breathing in a short, sharp and explosive manner. And you will not last very long when exercising if the breath is either too hard or too soft for particular activities that require a specific type of breathing style, such as for swimming or tennis.

The ultimate aim is to become so versatile with your breathing that you can use it in as many different ways as possible. Being able to adjust the softness and strength of your inhalation and exhalation will give you much more control over your breathing, such as when you are relaxing or exercising.

The breathing scale

Throughout this book, we will be referring to a scale from 1 to 10, which measures control and quality in breathing according to *volume* and *pace*.

Each number on the scale represents the volume (pitch)—1 being soft and delicate, 10 being hard and powerful; and the pace (speed)—1 being slow, 10 being fast.

1	Volume (V) = as low as possible Pace (P) = very slow and as long as possible
2	V and P slightly increase
3	
4	By this stage, there is a definite change in the volume and pace. The sound of the breath is a lot firmer and stronger. The volume and pace is starting to increase obviously.
5	A steady increase in V and P.
6	
7	
8	By 8 and 9 you are power breathing.
9	The breath is short, sharp and powerful.
10	The maximum—can be achieved only if you have an extremely strong diaphragm and excellent breathing skills.

BREATHING SCALE EXERCISE

Beginning at 1, gradually progress up to 10. At 1, breathe as if you have a feather on your palm and you have to inhale and exhale without moving it. At 10, you should be breathing your hardest, as if you were blowing out a hundred candles in one go.

THE RELAXATION BREATH

The relaxation breath is a throat breath on a scale of 2. It literally lays the foundation for good quality breathing. Firstly, do the exercise with your mouth slightly open, thereafter, through the nose. We will begin with gentle and extended breathing—so keep the level at 1 or 2.

We will work on the exhalation first. With mouth slightly open, inhale deeply and breathe out for as long as possible. Aim to keep the breath gentle and smooth from the beginning right until the end. Do this a few times until you feel confident with it.

Next, try it on the inhalation. Take particular care on the inhalation not to breathe too hard or too quickly.

Now repeat the same procedure, but through the nose only. Begin with the exhalation first. You might need extra time when attempting the inhalation. I strongly suggest that you practice the relaxation breath until you master it (see page 144 for more detail), making sure that the inhalation is at least almost as good as the exhalation.

THE POWER BREATH

Next we will try a powerful version of the relaxation breath. Again, start with the exhalation, keeping your mouth slightly open and relaxed, inhale deeply and then exhale as hard as you can through the mouth. Imagine you are on 10 on the scale with volume and pace. Now try to breathe out hard, but try to make the breath last longer, at around 7. Repeat for the inhalation.

Now go through the procedure again through the nose only. You may find it more difficult, and you might resort to sniffing. If so, reduce the level of the breath and begin at about 4 or 5, and gradually work your way up. You can do each stage properly only if you are predominately emphasizing the muscles of your throat rather than those of your nose. (See pages 115–116 for more detail.)

VARIATIONS

You should now begin to practice all of the exercises above, using the scale to help you achieve exactly what you want. Experiment with varying the scale by adjusting from one level to the next. Can you notice how involved the muscles of your throat and your diaphragm are when you adjust? And can you feel how much you need to increase the use and intensity of those muscles as you move up the scale, especially when dynamically power breathing? Have you realized how you can change the kind of breath produced simply by the volume and pace you choose.

With practice, you will become confident with your ability to pull in a large breath to the exact amount that you choose, and for much longer than what you are used to.

You can also breathe to various stages within one long breath. Begin at 1 and gradually go to 5, 7, down to 3, up to 8, etc. Think of the exercise like a singer hitting different notes, or changing the volume dial on your radio.

All these exercises show you the vast amount of variation there is when it comes to breathing. You could literally spend hours experimenting with all of them! Only by grasping these exercises can you become an all-around and adaptive breather. These exercises form the basis for you to work from. The important objective is that as a result, you learn to regulate your breath and also to adapt your breathing to any demand.

It is crucial to grasp this section on throat breathing. It is the first concept I teach both privately and to groups, and I consider it to be the most important. You need to develop the inhalation so it is as strong as the exhalation. Every aspect of breathing must be totally balanced—you should be able to inhale and exhale both softly and powerfully, quickly and slowly and for longer than you could normally. Without mastering basic throat breathing, you cannot move on to the next stages, so take your time and put the effort in now.

Breathing in components and emphasizing body parts

....

To build a strong foundation in breathing training, you must learn to breathe gently and slowly for long periods of time. You must also be able to breathe in intervals for a number of times within an extended breath. I call this the "component factor." Think of it as learning to crawl before you learn to walk. It is one of the most important lessons required in order to lengthen and control the breath. (It might sound difficult or confusing, but I have step-by-step instructions for you to follow.)

One of the biggest mistakes I see when people attempt to take a deep breath is breathing in too much, too soon, and with too much urgency—like a gasp! As mentioned, slow, lengthened breathing is the foundation that all other kinds of breathing techniques come from. If all you are capable of is taking your biggest breath in one quick burst, how will you ever lengthen your breath for times that it is needed, for example, when wanting to relax or for flexibility exercises?

I must clarify that the component exercises and learning how to lengthen your breath serve the purpose of training your breathing muscles and improving your breathing. You are not required to try to prolong your breath at any time other than during the breathing training session, or when you need a lengthened breath for a specific purpose. What I am suggesting here will ultimately help you achieve a good quality and relaxed breath. This chapter does not have anything to do with your natural quiet breathing, which you should simply allow to happen automatically.

When learning how to increase the length of your breath, you must combine small components (of breath) with an extra slow breathing pace. You must also move particular body parts used during respiration and not exaggerate movement of the shoulders or upper chest. The use of throat breathing is crucial, otherwise you will not be able to execute the exercise properly.

The following exercises require you to hold your breath to some degree, and it is important that you gain approval from your doctor before you attempt them.

SINGLE PAUSE EXERCISE

When you learned how to throat breathe, you learned to extend the "H" in "HA." This exercise continues on from there. Breathe only one "H" at a time with a slight pause in between. There is a count of one second for the "H" and one second for the pause:

H – H – H – H – H – H – H – H – H – H – H – H – H – H

Begin with the exhalation and keep going until you run out of breath. Now do the inhalation, and continue until you cannot breathe in any more. Repeat a couple of times.

DOUBLE PAUSE EXERCISE

This is the master exercise—one of the most important for lengthening your breath. This time, the count is for two seconds. Two "H"s and two pauses in between:

H H – – H H – – H H – – H H – – H H – – H H – – H H – – H H

Do the exhalation first, then the inhalation. In both instances, go for as long as possible until you reach the end of your breath. Repeat this exercise three or more times each. If you grasp this exercise now, you will find all of the breathing training much easier.

The above exercises are designed to prevent you from breathing too much, too soon and too quickly, which results in short, shallow breaths. When you are employing the component factor, you should only be concerned with inhaling one little bit of breath, and at the same time, moving the relevant body parts minutely. Another advantage of the component factor is that you can keep visualizing and refocusing exactly where you want the breath to go, so specifically aim for the diaphragm area (not the upper chest).

Regulating the breath with movement

Whether during exercise or breathing training, failing to properly regulate the breath as you move is one of the biggest faults with those who are inexperienced. Your body is programmed to synchronize your breath with movement, so it happens automatically. However, I want you to concentrate on breathing fully and evenly throughout the whole movement, rather than focusing on the beginning. If your breath and movement are out of alignment by even a small amount, it can influence overall performance. You will still be able to move and function, but if you want to achieve a high standard in exercise and breathing training, learning how to regulate the breath efficiently is a must. Professional athletes are extremely proficient at regulating their breathing, particularly for endurance sports. Once you master this ability, you will wonder how you ever exercised without it.

REGULATING EXERCISE—OPEN/CLOSE FIST

1 Begin with your hand out flat. Slowly and smoothly close your hand to make a fist and then slowly open it again back to the starting position. This time, we will do the same movement and match it with our breathing. So with hand out flat, take a nice deep breath in. From the exact moment you begin to close your fist, also begin to exhale. The aim is to finish your exhalation precisely as your hand becomes a closed fist.

2 Next, open the hand and inhale at the same time. Once again, begin the inhalation the exact moment you begin to open your hand. The aim is to have inhaled as much as you can by the time the hand is fully opened and flat.

3 Now repeat the same exercise (parts 1 and 2) to extremes. Do it as slowly as you possibly can, then as quickly as possible.

REGULATING EXERCISE—UP/DOWN ARM

1 Stand (or sit if you cannot stand) with hands by your side. Move your arm upward away from your body and then back to starting position.

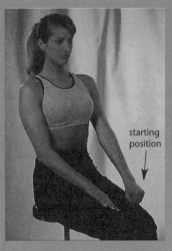
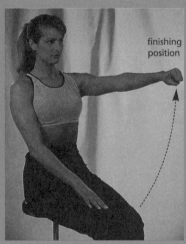

starting position

finishing position

2 Do the same movement but this time regulate your breathing, the same as you did with the open/close fist exercise above. The movement of the arm going upward is the most difficult part of the exercise. There is a tendency to breathe in

too much at the beginning of the movement, and run out of breath toward the end of the final movement.

3 Repeat the exercise going as slowly as you can, then as fast as you can. Make sure both the arm and breath begin and finish *exactly* at the same time.

The aim is to make sure your breath is consistent throughout the whole movement, including the last part. You have done it correctly when the inhalation and the exhalation sound the same throughout the whole movement from beginning to end. The sound should be audible from beginning to end, with a sense of strength and smoothness about it.

Using your imagination to emphasize different body parts

The imagination is a powerful tool, and it can be used in breathing training to help "emphasize" specific body parts. Singing teachers use visualization in this way also, in order to achieve certain results. When I say "emphasizing specific body parts," I should point out that no muscle really does move in isolation. For example, if you lift a finger, it may look like only that particular finger is moving, but in fact many other muscles of the hand and arm were also involved. However, using your imagination to visualize only that particular finger moving can help you to hone in on those specific muscles and to minimize the effect on the surrounding ones.

In order to become really proficient with your breathing, you will need to learn how to hone in on one or more muscles used for the respiration process. For example, I might say to move only the diaphragm without moving any other body part and only toward the end of the breath, move the abdomen. The reality is that both the abdomen and chest are involved whenever the diaphragm moves, but you should imagine that you are working the diaphragm only, until another body part is needed. By mentally emphasizing particular muscles, you can control which muscles you predominately use. And in this way you can learn to use different types of breathing, such as diaphragmatic and power breathing.

When I demonstrate how to move the diaphragm and rib cage without an obvious movement from the upper chest, I am often greeted with amazement, and am asked, "How could I possibly do that?" Much to their surprise, most people do end up doing to a greater or lesser degree what they initially thought was impossible. Everyone can lean how to focus on specific body parts and muscles used during the respiratory process. I have even witnessed elderly people with seemingly immovable rib cages achieve amazing results.

How is it possible to emphasize different body parts?

You already know how to emphasize different parts of your body. Keep your left arm and hand absolutely still as you open and close the right hand. Is that difficult? You commanded one part of your body to keep still while instructing another part to move. Your brain gave the instruction to a specific body part to move in isolation while the rest of the hand remained still. Your conscious mind does not need to know exactly how this phenomenon takes place. We are internally programmed to know how to do this, so that when the mind gives the instruction, the body automatically obeys and responds.

As a baby, you might not have been able to move and control specific body parts, but as a result of seeing others and practicing, you were eventually able to. By constantly practicing, you slowly improved and eventually sharpened your body's ability to respond to what you consciously asked of it. If you have never had any form of breathing training, you are also in the learning stage of being able to fully control different parts of your body relevant to controlled breathing.

If you are in the learning stage, you will need to practice and be patient until the process becomes easy. And it will become second nature if you practice regularly and trust the innate wisdom of the human body. You should mentally keep giving the instruction and trust that your body will sooner or later respond. Even if at first the response is a small one, it will lay the foundation for the muscles to be controlled and strengthened.

AWARENESS EXERCISE

Place your fingertips on your belly button. As you breathe in, mentally instruct the belly button to go outward. Next breathe out, and with your fingers push your belly button inward toward your spine. Repeat a few times until you can do it on mental command alone without the use of your fingers on the belly button. It may feel awkward and difficult at first, but it will become easy quite quickly.

EXERCISES TO EMPHASIZE MUSCLES AND BODY MOVEMENTS

You need to learn how to move the rib cage without an exaggerated movement of the shoulders, upper chest and abdomen, and without dropping the chest. You also need to learn how to minimize movement of the abdomen while moving the rib cage through a full range of movement inward and outward—most people can master it after a bit of practice.

1 First do this exercise lying down. Place hands on the abdomen and as you exhale, use your hands to push the abdomen area upward and inward toward

the spine. Even though you will be breathing in and out, keep the abdomen in this exact position because, more than any other way, it will give you freedom to work with the rib cage and diaphragm. With small, controlled movements, move your rib cage inward and outward. Make the inhalation and exhalation movements both equal in duration. Do you sense that the upper chest and shoulders are moving too much? If so, consider whether:

- you are sniff breathing instead of throat breathing.

- you are predominately emphasizing the upper chest muscles rather than the diaphragm.

- your upper chest was dropped to begin with instead of up and open.

- you have relaxed the abdomen too much and the ribs have dropped downward.

The rib cage can be moved inward without the upper chest dropping. Can you finish an exhale so that the rib cage and chest look like the shape of a barrel, rather than a deflated tire? The diaphragm must be emphasized and employed to achieve this rounded look, along with good upright posture. Let the diaphragm control the movement and lead the way, rather than your shoulders and the muscles of your upper chest.

Only when you have mastered stage one, should you go on to stage two. You might need to stay with stage one for quite some time, while others, who are experienced at specialized forms of breathing, might grasp controlling the diaphragm straight away. It doesn't matter how long it takes. What matters is that you must learn how to do this before you move on. Ultimately, this skill gives you an incredible amount of control and allows you to fine-tune your breathing apparatus.

2 Having mastered the small movements in stage one, begin to very slowly increase the inward and outward movement of the ribs. When increasing, be aware that you might begin to slip into old habits that no longer serve you. Be careful that you don't:

- breathe too much or too hard.

- breathe too fast or abruptly.

- lift or drop your upper chest.

- obviously move your shoulders upward or downward.

Begin by increasing the movement by twice as much as you did in stage one. Then keep increasing the duration for as long as you can while maintaining the correct posture and technique.

Posture

Proper posture is essential for good quality breathing. Drooping, rounded shoulders cause the chest to drop downward, which prevents us from breathing fully because the diaphragm and lungs are cramped. However, when you keep the chest high, the diaphragm, ribs and abdominal muscles are free to move without inhibition.

Many health problems begin with poor posture. Most back and neck pain is a result of slack or tense muscles, and incorrect posture that has thrown the body out of alignment. Internal sluggishness may be due to cramped internal organs caused by slouching. Therefore, I cannot stress enough how important good posture is. I would encourage you to visit a chiropractor or an osteopath to have yours checked, particularly if you suffer from any kind of back or neck problems.

You could also try the Alexander Technique, which is a process of physical re-education concerned with changing the way you use your body as a whole. Instructors teach awareness through movement (via the mind/body connection) and the "unlearning" of bad postural habits. F. Matthias Alexander was an actor from Tasmania who developed the technique in order to project his voice more effectively on stage. However, the results he began to find astounded him so much that he eventually gave up the stage and dedicated his life to developing and teaching the technique around the world. It is still very popular today with actors, musicians and singers, as well as people with back, neck and other muscular-skeletal problems. I learned the Alexander Technique 13 years ago, and to this day, I still use the basic principles to help me with my posture. Books are available on the subject, but nothing can compare with one-on-one sessions with a trained instructor.

In order to breathe fully, you should be aware of the following points with regard to your posture (particularly when you are doing breathing training):

1. The back of your neck should be lengthened, with your chin toward your chest. If your head is out of alignment by being either too far forward or back, tilt your chin slightly downward and elongate your neck.

2. Your upper chest should be open and lengthened in a relaxed manner. You are standing incorrectly if your chest looks and/or feels sunken.

3. Your shoulders need to be up and back in a relaxed manner, in their natural position. You are standing incorrectly if your shoulders hang forward, or if they are elevated because of too much tension.

4. The whole rib cage should have an "openness" about it. Aim to make the distance from your hips to your armpits as elongated as possible.

5. The position of the diaphragm must be high and relaxed. You cannot detect this visually, so use your mental awareness. You can use your fingers to try to feel the position of the diaphragm muscle and whether or not it is relaxed.

CORRECT POSTURE FOR BREATHING

Now let's begin the first exercise. Stand or kneel in front of a mirror. Do not sit unless you have an injury. You need to be bare-chested or wearing a sports top, as you need to see how the muscles move beneath the skin. Now assess your posture. Take your time.

Before you get started, it is important to breathe in and out whenever you need to, particularly if you feel light-headed or unusual in any way, regardless of what the instructions say.

Begin by breathing in, long and deep, as much as you can, but without any strain or struggle. At the top of this inhalation, hold your breath for a moment and assess your posture. Take a mental note of how you look and feel in this posture, so that you can refer to it in the future. You should feel a real sense of openness and freedom. From now on, I will refer to this as the position of "perfect posture."

Imagine a champion athlete you admire, and then visualize a person lacking in confidence. The biggest visual indication of their character—whether weak or powerful—is how they hold themselves. See for yourself how you feel when you are collapsed in a poor posture; then lift yourself up and put yourself in an up-and-open correct posture. Your mental state changes automatically, and you feel more positive, confident and uplifted.

You will also notice how much easier it is to breathe in this posture. Once your spine and the appropriate muscles are strengthened and kept in their appropriate place, correct posture will become much easier for you to maintain. So keep checking yourself regularly throughout the day, adjusting and correcting as necessary. Persist in doing this until you feel comfortable in an upright position. And when you do, you will find you have improved breathing, improved internal health and mental well-being, and all your physical actions will be easier to perform.

INCORRECT POSTURE
INHALATION   EXHALATION

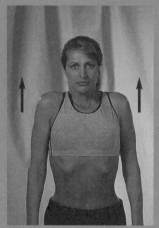 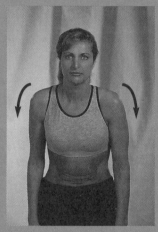

Shoulders and upper chest are raised upward.

Shoulders and upper chest drop and roll forward.

CORRECT POSTURE
INHALATION   EXHALATION

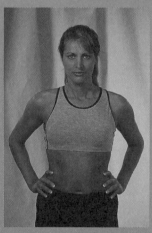 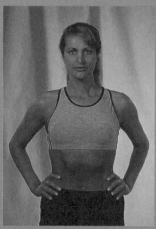

Check each of the points on pages 64–65, from one to five, to see if you have perfect posture. Not only is this how you should ideally hold yourself most of the time, this is also the established posture for the inhalation and exhalation. Even when you are at the end of your exhalation, the whole zone 1 area should be the same as you see it now at the peak of your inhalation. You should not allow your shoulders to droop or your chest to sink at any time. Only the rib cage and abdominal area should move. It is crucial that every part of zone 1 be kept still.

OPENING THE CHEST

Imagine the base of your upper spine and lift your sternum up, as if reaching for the sky. At the same time, keep your chin pointing toward your chest and your neck lengthened. Now relax and lengthen your shoulders, which will open your chest up even more. It will allow you to be freer and to lift your sternum even higher.

MEASURE UP!

You can use a measuring tape to help you feel what the correct posture should be. (You may need someone to help you.) Secure a measuring tape around your upper chest, in line with your armpits. Inhale deeply and see what the measurement is at this point. Now when you exhale, your chest should not change structure, and the measurement should hardly change either. *Your chest should continue to grip the tape as you exhale.* If it is not, you are allowing your chest to drop and not working your diaphragm and rib cage enough. Aim to breathe out so that the upper chest is constantly gripping the measuring tape enabling you to keep the chest up, open and full throughout the exercise. When you achieve this, mentally capture in your mind what this feels and looks like.

This is one of the best exercises to help you learn how your upper chest needs to be when practicing good quality breathing. You will need to use this open upper chest posture constantly throughout the training in this book. Repeat this exercise as many times as you feel you need to until you know you are doing it properly according to the measure on the tape.

CORRECT POSTURE FOR BREATHING— LYING DOWN

What you have just done standing, you will now do lying down, in order to learn what constitutes proper posture in any position. Lying down gives you the advantage of allowing you to be totally supported by the floor. On the other hand, you cannot see yourself as you could when you were standing in front of the mirror. So you need to use your inner awareness to visualize how you look. (It would be helpful if you could ask someone to check you. If they do not know anything at all about proper posture, they can read the checklist on pages 64–65.)

INCORRECT POSTURE   CORRECT POSTURE

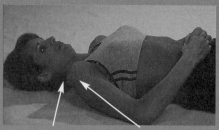
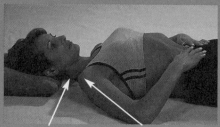

The neck is cramped.   Shoulders are too   Neck is relaxed and   Shoulders are flat on
                        high off the floor.   lengthened.   the floor.

Lie down and arrange yourself so you feel comfortable. Make sure your chin is in the direction of your chest and that your neck is lengthened. Are your shoulders widened and evenly spread out on the floor? If not, adjust yourself so they are. If you feel tension anywhere, try to relax that area.

Inhale deeply without strain or struggle. Simply inhale fully and gently hold the breath. Once again, ask yourself the same questions you did in front of the mirror: How do you feel at the top of your inhalation? What is your mental state? Do you feel mentally open or closed? How do you feel physically? Do you feel open and free or closed? You should feel free and open mentally and physically, with perfect posture in a lying down position. Again, commit this feeling to memory, as you will need to use it every time you practice good quality breathing. Do the exercise as many times as you need to in order to grasp it.

Here are some exercises that will help you to maintain perfect posture at all times, in particular during breathing training. This requires a lot of conscious effort in the beginning, until it becomes second nature. Do these exercises in front of a mirror first and then on the floor.

CORRECT POSTURE FOR EXHALATION— BASIC EXERCISE

Inhale nicely and deeply, and exhale for only two seconds then pause. Do you still have the same posture as when you started? If you have dropped your upper chest even a little, then the rest of your exhalation will not work, and you should start from the beginning again. Exhale another small breath. You should notice only a bit of a difference with your ribs moving inward and your belly button toward your spine. If your upper chest has moved at all, then you have failed and should start again. The ideal is to reach the end of your exhalation and still have perfect posture.

When you are on the floor, make sure your shoulders stay pinned flat against the floor as much as possible. Your ribs should have moved in toward each other, but still have an "openness" about them. If this is so, then you have held your posture correctly. Keep breathing out for two then hold for two until you reach the end of your breath. The aim is to finish exhaling without moving zone 1 at all. When you have completed this exercise on the floor, you are ready to try the advanced version.

ADVANCED EXERCISE

This time, aim for the breath to be one long, smooth and continuous exhalation—like air being released from a tire—without pausing. Breathe in to the top of your inhalation and then breathe out slowly in one continuous flow. By the time you reach the end of your exhalation, zone 1 should not have moved. If you have not done it properly, then you need to practice until it is correct.

Here's a tip: *do not try to deliberately tighten the abdominal muscles and the diaphragm area until the very end of the exhalation.* If you tighten the abdominal muscles and diaphragm area too soon—common faults—then the chest will automatically drop no matter how hard you try to keep it up.

Do not give up! Learn to relax your abdominal muscles and your diaphragm, and this will help to move them upward. The more you concentrate on keeping your shoulders still and pinned to the floor and your breastbone lifted high even as you are exhaling, the easier it will be to keep the upper chest from dropping. Also, imagine something is keeping your upper chest held high and open, like an imaginary jack inside your chest.

CORRECT POSTURE FOR INHALATION—
BASIC EXERCISE

To control the inhalation so that you can breathe long and deep, you need to be careful not to emphasize the upper chest area at all. There is a common tendency when using the sniff breath to lift and overexpand the upper chest—like a soldier. The task in this exercise is to make sure that zone 1 stays reasonably still and to emphasize zone 2 only—that is, to move mainly the lower ribs.

Stand in front of a mirror, as bare-chested as possible. The starting point of the exercise is at the end of the exhalation. Make sure you have perfect posture even after you have completely exhaled. Inhale only for two seconds, making sure that the diaphragm area is the focal point. Check to see that the upper chest doesn't expand. Keep inhaling for two-second components of breath. Check your shoulders. If they have become tense and have moved upward, then you have inhaled incorrectly. You must not move any part in zone 1. Start again and continue until you get it right.

The mirror is perfect for this exercise because you can instantly see if there is any movement in the shoulders and upper chest. For this reason, mirror work is a must for everyone, especially in the beginning stages. It is something I still occasionally do just as a periodic check.

ADVANCED EXERCISE

Completely exhale and make sure you have perfect posture. Begin by slowly breathing in one long continuous inhalation. Keep checking that your shoulders are relaxed and not lifting upward. Tip: you must keep your neck lengthened at all times, keeping your chin toward your chest.

Try the exercise again, aiming not to move zone 1 at all or at least to a minimum. If you are having difficulty getting it right, you may even wish to go back to the basic exercise again to get on the right track. Only when you can do it correctly should you move on to the advanced exercise. Practice the exercise lying down as well.

FINE-TUNING EXERCISE

Finally, to fine-tune this section is to do both the inhalation and the exhalation as one uninterrupted breath without any pausing. Inhale in one long continuous breath and then one long continuous exhalation. Check that your whole posture is correct as you are breathing in and out. Do the exercise in front of the mirror and on the floor. Again, make sure the upper chest is not dropping and lifting as you breathe in and out. If you can do the exercise without greatly moving any part of zone 1 and you can see your ribs moving inward and outward (rather than up and down) and your abdomen moving upward and downward, then you have achieved perfect posture. This is an essential stage to master before you can go on to improve your breathing. From now on, your ability to breathe fully and properly will be much easier.

Flexibility and stretching

Apart from a few lucky naturally flexible people and the people who work hard at staying flexible, almost everyone at times complains about feeling stiff! Stretching improves performance, joint stability and joint range of motion and reduces the risk of injury. Sports people stretch various muscle groups after an initial warmup, which is advisable for everybody. Stretching is usually slow and held for eight to twelve seconds or longer. I believe in aiming to achieve flexibility for your whole body, but this chapter will focus more on the abdomen, chest and neck area in reference to better breathing.

If you breathe inappropriately and assume an incorrect posture, there will be an automatic resistance like a tight band around the chest area. If you want to breathe deeply, the breath needs room to move. Fortunately, it is a problem that can be solved. All you need to do is "let go" of the tension in the neck, chest and respiratory muscles, stop overusing the chest and shoulders unnecessarily, and consciously use the diaphragm and abdomen in a more relaxed manner.

Your skeletal muscles will respond to your conscious instructions. So by bringing your awareness to the tension developed in your muscles, you can then allow the tightness to be released by simply suggesting that the muscles relax as you slowly and deeply exhale. I have seen this happen time and time again, so rest assured it is possible, even if you are inflexible to begin with.

The chest and rib cage area needs to be opened up because you will not be able to fully lengthen your breath if the relevant muscles are stiff. Also, as your breathing increases, you will need to expand your chest and rib cage more, so there is space for the increased volume of breath to move in.

Flexibility and correct posture allow the diaphragm, rib cage and abdomen to move freely and through a full range of motion inward and outward. When we allow the ribs to move fully, we use more of our lung capacity, giving the lungs a thorough work out.

The following body parts can inhibit relaxed deep breathing when they are tense:

- face and tongue
- throat and neck
- shoulders and upper chest area

- diaphragm and rib cage
- abdominal muscles

  Some other factors that interfere with relaxed deep breathing include:

- lifting and heaving the shoulders, which causes unnecessary tension in the neck, chest and upper back area.
- restriction in the upper chest, which forces the shoulders to droop forward, and also restricts full movement of the diaphragm.
- a tight, stiff diaphragm, which cannot produce maximal power during forceful contractions.
- overly tight intercostal muscles, which interfere with the rib cage's fully opening and closing in an unrestricted manner.
- tensed abdominal muscles that prevent full movement of the diaphragm and restrict total completion of a lengthened breath.

Bear in mind that you may have some or all of the above faults, yet you may still be breathing efficiently naturally. The above factors refer specifically to relaxed deep breathing. So apart from the diaphragm and abdomen not being able to fully relax, if muscles around the chest and rib cage are also too tight, the restrictions will inhibit you from taking your deepest relaxation breath.

What can be done?

- Tension should be released in relevant muscles, in particular: upper chest, diaphragm and abdominal muscles.
- All muscles involved in respiration should be relaxed.
- The rib cage and lungs need to be expanded and opened up as much as possible.
- The diaphragm should be strengthened.

One of the biggest problems I see is locked-in tension in the abdomen and diaphragm muscle and the inability to let that tension go. The positive news is that as a result of relaxed and lengthened breathing, the abdomen, diaphragm and lungs work as a unit to produce a good quality breath. In order to breathe deeply, all the respiratory muscles must be completely relaxed. Especially in the learning stage, muscle relaxation must happen by conscious instruction each step of the way. The more relaxed and toned all these muscles are, the easier it is to breathe fully. By incorporating every aspect required in the act of breathing deeply, the whole breathing apparatus will be able to function with greater ease and with optimal versatility.

The most important points to remember when doing lengthened inhaling and exhaling are:

- The abdomen and diaphragm must be completely relaxed throughout most of the breath in order to consciously move them.

- You must also be able to tighten the abdomen and the diaphragm when appropriate.

You improve your flexibility for breathing by:

- learning how to consciously control the abdominal muscles, so that you can relax and tighten them as easily as you can control making a fist and relaxing it again.
- taking a longer breath slowly and deeply to effectively relax all muscles involved in breathing.
- improving posture and flexibility in zones 1, 2 and 3.
- massaging the tense muscles that are involved, directly or indirectly, in the act of breathing.

As you increase your breathing capacity and improve your posture, you will be surprised at the difference you will feel. A tense, sunken chest will be a thing of the past. Your diaphragm and ribs will have a full range of movement where they were previously restricted. This will allow you to breathe with ease and total freedom without feeling limited and constricted.

If you are not very flexible, you are not alone. Most people complain of being inflexible, but, in particular, men commonly complain to me that they feel unbearably tight and restricted. Rib cage changes occur with age, and I have found men aged 50 plus tend to experience the most difficulty learning how to release tension in that whole area. Women who are inflexible tend to respond quicker and find it easier to move their rib cage. In general, unless you keep practicing flexibility exercises, the older you are, the more inflexible you are.

The good news is that despite your age, sex and level of flexibility, you can improve. Even the most stubborn rib cages will finally loosen up and become more flexible. The fact is that it may take some people longer than others to achieve basic flexibility, but if you work at it, you'll get there in the end.

I can recall the ecstatic response of some men I have trained who finally achieved some movement with their stiff ribs. As a result of this newfound freedom, many of them would leave the session with excitement saying, "I feel like a kid again," or "I feel like a new man!" I couldn't help but share their enthusiasm.

Initially, I suggest you spend some extra time on loosening up. If you can do some flexibility exercises for 5 to 15 minutes every day for a month, you will see a vast improvement. Then, you will only need a few minutes a day to open the chest area up. Once you achieve a basic level of flexibility, it is easy to maintain it.

Most people don't like to stretch their bodies—usually because they feel so stiff! It is a common habit to hold on to the breath when stretching, which makes the whole process difficult and painful. In actual fact, you are stretching incorrectly if it hurts too much. Stretching to improve your flexibility can be a pleasant experience when performed properly.

Holding on to your breath when you do stretching exercises causes pain because the muscle tightens instead of relaxing. Many people avoid stretching because it is too painful. As you release the built-up tension in your body and learn to breathe and stretch properly, you will actually start to look forward to flexibility exercises because they make you feel taller and more relaxed throughout your body.

By stretching a muscle, you help to lengthen and relax it and help to avoid injury. If you choose not to stretch your whole body, then at the very least stretch your rib cage area. Whether you are young or old, male or female, it is worth the time and effort to keep the chest and rib cage area as flexible as possible in order to breathe more freely.

I suggest doing the flexibility exercises for your whole chest area first thing in the morning. Although any time is good, stretching before you start the day gets you off to a good start. Try committing yourself to stretching your whole chest area for a month. Once it becomes a habit, you will wonder how you ever started your day without it. The flexibility exercises are also invaluable before exercising.

If you continue stretching, you can actually change the structure of your posture. As you release the tension and allow your muscles to loosen up from being tight, they will allow your posture to be in its natural, upright position instead of pulling inward and drooping forward. You will begin to notice that this new improved posture will be your new natural way of holding your body all the time. Because the appropriate muscles have lengthened, it will not be a strain—in fact, if you put a bit of effort in at the beginning, you will eventually find that being in an incorrect posture probably will be more of a strain.

The stretching routine

This stretching routine is specially designed to open up the rib cage and chest area. Not only can the exercises help you breathe better, but gradually they will improve your posture, if you do them regularly. The routine will take you about 10 minutes to complete. If you are pressed for time, you can choose the two most important ones (horizontal and vertical stretches, pages 76–77) and do them every day. If you are inflexible, I suggest you practice all of the exercises for a while, at least until you have loosened up a little.

The most important point when you are stretching is to *always breathe out slowly and deeply when lengthening a muscle and releasing the tightness.*

Deeply inhale on the passive part of the stretch, and exhale slowly on the active part. If your exhalation finishes before the duration of your stretch, then *stop moving at that point, inhale deeply, and then continue stretching. Don't push yourself to keep stretching, even though the breath has finished.* For difficult stretches, you may need to repeat this procedure a few times within the one stretch.

THE TENSION CHECK

Before you begin stretching (and before breathing training), you should do the *tension check*—a simple process that makes you aware of where in your body you are holding on to tension. Stand or sit still and mentally scan your body, noting the areas that are tight or stiff. The shoulders and neck are tense in many people. Check particularly the following body parts:

- eyes, jaw and neck
- shoulders
- chest
- stomach area
- back: upper, middle and lower
- legs and feet

This only needs to take a minute or two. Once you become more in tune with your body, you will instantly know when you are holding on to tension. This then gives you the opportunity to release it, rather than hold it. So where did you detect your problem areas? Can you loosen up those areas a bit by massaging them or moving a bit? Do whatever you need to release a bit of the tightness. The more relaxed you are before you stretch and breathe deeply, the easier it will be to do everything.

It is very important that you be patient with the stretching exercises. Even if you do the first stages for a long time, you will still gain enormous benefits. The aim is to stretch, not to force the end result.

Stretches for greater flexibility

Please check with an exercise physiologist or physiotherapist before attempting these stretches. Everyone should do an initial warmup before beginning stretching exercises.

The stretches will be divided into two groups. Stage 1 is for those of you who are not very flexible and feel stretching is a painful process. Stage 2 is for people who are extremely flexible and have no problem stretching. Even if you are flexible, still be very cautious if you have not done these particular stretches.

Most people will begin with stage 1 and should stay at this level until their muscles have completely relaxed and lengthened. You may feel you always need to stay on this level. This is perfectly acceptable as most people have great difficulty with flexibility, particularly elderly people, many men and muscle-bound athletes.

IMAGERY EXERCISE

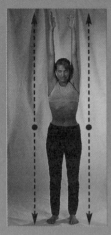

Before you get started, I want you to try this imagery exercise. While you stretch your arms up high, imagine you have an arrow starting at your belly button going toward the ground and another starting at your belly button and reaching toward the sky. This will help you to lengthen as much as you can throughout the exercise, but keep a solid grounding at the same time (which is the most effective way to stretch).

If you have time to do only a couple of stretches, do the first two exercises—the horizontal stretch and the vertical stretch. The first is the best stretch of them all in my opinion and should be performed daily. Even stretching every second day is effective and better than doing nothing at all.

Reminder: only use deep throat breathing. Keep your breath flowing and moving throughout the whole procedure. Inhale deeply before you stretch, and very importantly, the exhalation should be very long and slow as you move and stretch.

HORIZONTAL STRETCH

STAGE 1 AND 2

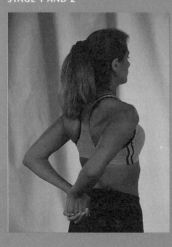

This effectively stretches the muscles of the chest, arms and around the rib cage.

Stage 1

1 Stand evenly on both feet. Lift your sternum right up, making sure your chin is toward the ground and your neck is relaxed and lengthened. Put your arms behind your back and clasp your hands so that your palms are facing toward each other and your fingers are intertwined. Hold for a few seconds at a time.

2 As you loosen up, aim to touch your shoulder blades together and gradually straighten your arms as much as you can without feeling any strain from your arms or chest.

STAGE 1 AND 2

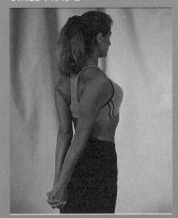

STAGE 2 ONLY

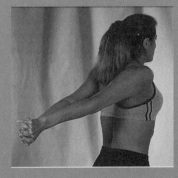

Stage 2

1 If you are really flexible, press your palms together so that the heels of the palms are firmly pressing against each other. Breathe out and straighten your arms as much as possible. The ultimate stretch is to have your arms really straight and at the same time, turn the elbows inward so that they are facing each other. Only when you can do all this with ease should you move on to the next step.

2 Breathe in first without moving. With your arms straight and your elbows inward, slowly move your hands up as you exhale. Be sure that the heels of the palms stay together the whole time, even as you move upward. If you are hurting too much at any point, you have moved upward too far and need to drop your hands to a more bearable level, at which you can still feel the stretch. When you are at the right level, stop and hold that position for a while so that the chest muscles can lengthen and loosen up. Keep gently throat breathing in and out as you hold. Slowly come out of it as you exhale.

VERTICAL STRETCH

Stage 1

1 Stretch your right arm high above your head so that your elbow is high above your head and stretch your left arm toward the ground. Breathing out, bring your right arm downward in a semi-circle on to the shoulder blade with the palm facing downward. Breathe in, then breathe out again, this time bringing your left arm upward as far as you comfortably can, making sure the palm is facing outward.

2 For most of you, there will be a gap. (You may use a belt to help bridge the distance until you become more flexible.) Hold for a little while, breathing long, slow and deep. Carefully and slowly undo yourself and repeat on the other side. You will find that one side is more difficult to stretch than the other. This is common and you should work more on your tighter side in order to make both sides even.

STAGE 1 AND 2

STAGE 1 AND 2

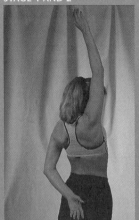 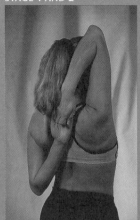

Stage 2

Follow step 1 as outlined above, but make sure you stretch your right arm as high as possible and use the elbow as a pivot point when bringing it downward. If you are flexible, there should not be a gap and you should be able to comfortably grasp the left hand as it is moving upward. Aim to move the right hand down into the left as much as possible. Repeat on the other side.

SIDE-BEND STRETCH

STAGE 1

STAGE 1

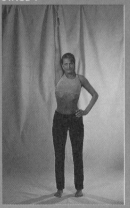 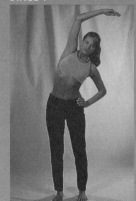

1 Stretch with your right arm, making sure your elbow is high above your head. At the same time, make sure your feet are grounded and are firmly pressing into the floor. Keep lengthening your torso and try to continually maintain that length during the stretch.

2 Breathe in, and with your left hand, take hold of your right arm just underneath your elbow. Breathe out and stretch upward even more, keeping your feet firmly pressed to the floor.

3 Breathe in deeply, then breathe out, bending over to your left. Bend only a little bit, but keep lengthening and stretching your arm and your torso as you bend. Make sure you don't squash your torso as you bend over. Your arm should stay in line with your ear the whole time. Hold for as long as you feel comfortable. Breathe in as you start to move back to the starting position. Make sure you are moving very slowly and carefully. Continually lengthen your arm and torso as you move upward. Repeat on the other side.

Stage 2
Repeat the same procedure as above, but bend sideways a bit more, making sure your arm is always in line with your ear. Also make sure that your body is in perfect alignment the whole time and that you do not lean forward or backward at any time.

STICK STRETCH

You will need a reasonably long stick, for example a broomstick. (You may do this with a long belt or rope if you do not have a stick, but they will not be as effective.) You will need a stick that is long enough for you to spread your arms across quite wide, particularly if you are not very flexible. You can decrease the distance as your flexibility improves.

STAGE 1 AND 2 STAGE 1 AND 2

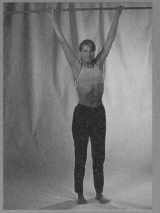 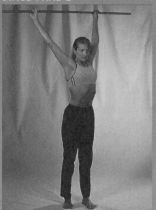

1 To begin, stand evenly on both feet, shoulder width apart. Inhale as you lift yourself up, stretching your arms and torso. Use the stick to really lengthen your body upward and keep your feet firmly on the ground at the same time. Remember the two-arrows concept and allow this to help you stretch even more.

Also, aim to lift your elbows way above your head. Take advantage of this openness and really B-R-E-A-T-H-E deeply as much as you possibly can while in this position. After a few breaths, exhale as you bring the stick down, but see if you can keep the torso lengthened even when you have returned to the starting position.

Stage 2
STAGE 2 ONLY

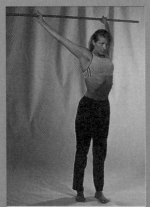

If you are flexible, you will be able to put your arms upward as above, but also backward. Be careful when you perform this backward move. Continue lengthening your arms and stretch them outward, even as you stretch them back over your head. Inhale before you move and exhale as you stretch back and up. (Stop and inhale and exhale a few times if you cannot do the whole movement on one exhalation.)

You must keep your arms straight the whole time. As your flexibility increases, you will gradually be able to comfortably go back further. When you have stretched back as far as you can, lift your sternum and take advantage of the openness and breathe fully and deeply. Before returning to the starting position, inhale first. Then exhale as you come out of it, still stretching upward and outward with your arms until you return to the original position. See if you can maintain the length of your torso even when you have finished.

FORWARD-BEND STRETCH

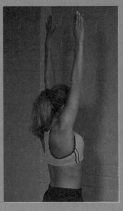
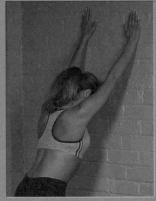

If you have a bad back or neck, I suggest you skip this stretch. Whether you are a beginner or more advanced, you should constantly make sure you are maintaining good form and proper posture throughout this stretch and that your knees remain bent.

Stage 1

Stand at arm's distance from a wall with feet shoulder width apart. Inhale as you stretch your arms upward as high as they can go. Bend your knees slightly and exhale as you slowly move and lean toward the wall, keeping your arms in line with your ears. Move until you touch the wall and hold that position for a few breaths. Use the angle you are in and the strength of the wall to really stretch your arms. Keep breathing deeply as you are stretching. To come out of this position, really bend your knees and fully inhale as you return to the starting position.

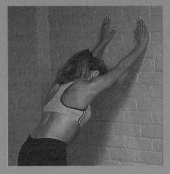

Stage 2

Aim to lean a little bit lower than you did in stage 1. The instructions are the same as above, but you will have more of a distance to cover, therefore making it more difficult. You must have a strong back in order to do this advanced stage.

BACKWARD-PRAYER STRETCH

Stage 2 only

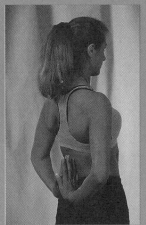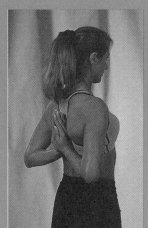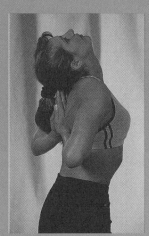

This should be attempted only by very flexible people, as it is quite difficult. Place both hands behind you with your fingertips toward your spine. Next, place your two small fingers flat further up on your spine. Bring your shoulders and shoulder blades inward as much as you can before going on to the next stage.

Your flexibility will determine how much you can move your hands up your spine. The ideal is to reach your hands upward to a point where you can comfortably drop your head back to touch your fingertips. (I did say it was difficult!)

Massage

Massage can be used all over the body for relaxation. It is also particularly good as part of breathing training because it can loosen up the muscles of the neck, shoulders, chest, back, rib cage area, rim of the diaphragm and the abdomen. While all muscles need attention, the most important areas to work on for better breathing are the rim of the diaphragm and the whole abdominal area.

Massage increases blood flow to the muscles and helps to release tension in tight, stiff muscles. It is also stimulating for muscles that have been inactive and is good for relieving tenderness.

At first you will probably feel a little soreness or tenderness when you touch certain body parts. This proves even more that you have locked-in tension that needs to be released.

As you release this tension, you will not find the same area painful or tender to touch—although it might take a little while to get to this ideal stage if you have been tight for a number of years. So patience is required.

It is best to gently massage your tender areas once or twice a week until the soreness is gone. Then do it occasionally as maintenance. You can massage any time you like, as long as you have an empty stomach.

There are three different options on how to approach massage: one, self-massage; two, call in the professionals; three, ask another person to help.

How to self-massage

I suggest you begin with self-massage. It will give you a deeper understanding of where and why you feel constricted with your breathing and where you hold tension within your body.

For your best results, relax and breathe out when a muscle is being massaged, especially if it feels sore. While your aim is to release the tension, do as much as you can handle without too much force or pressure.

The neck and shoulders

Begin by lying on your back and making yourself as comfortable as you can. Take a few deep relaxing breaths. After a few breaths, begin to become aware of where you feel the most tension. Neck and shoulders are the most common problem areas, so begin by gently massaging them, including the back of the shoulders.

Ribs and diaphragm

Most people find that these areas are quite tender, so take it very easy, especially the first time. Slowly and gently rub the space between each rib (intercostal muscles), from the breastbone right to the end of the rib. Then work the diaphragm area in a general way by pressing the balls of your fingers along the line of the rim of the diaphragm where the floating ribs are attached at the bottom of your rib cage.

Abdominal massage

The abdominal muscles go all the way from the pelvic bone right up to the sternum and lower rib cage. Lengthen and soften your exhalation, and as you do, dig as deep as you can without hurting yourself. Work all parts of the abdominal area, especially the middle section.

I also highly recommend professional massage. This is an incredibly effective way of releasing years of built up tension in the muscles. The advantage of having a professional massage is that you will be able to totally relax, and the masseur can properly access muscles that you or somebody inexperienced cannot.

Whether you are massaging yourself or another person is doing it for you, take note of where your problem areas are, and work on them slowly over a period of time. Remember that it may take many months for you to completely release tension that has been locked in the muscles for years.

How to give somebody else a massage of the respiratory muscles

Fifteen to 30 minutes is sufficient time to cover the whole respiratory area. Basic therapeutic and remedial massage techniques are used. The pressure is important. Too little pressure will not release the tension. Too much will cause an automatic reaction to tighten up, which negates the effect of relaxation needed. Be especially aware of too much pressure for females as they tend to be more fragile and tender, especially when elderly. Men, however, tend to be more muscular, so you might be able to apply more pressure. Regardless of sex or age, check with the person as you go along that the pressure is acceptable, especially if it is the first time.

1. First, have the person lie on his or her back on a table and make sure he or she is comfortable and warm.

2. Gently rub the neck, shoulders and upper chest area to help release some of the tension.

3. Work fingers along the ridges between the individual rib cage cartilages. In order to massage the rim of the diaphragm, use the thumbs to tuck under the sternum area and apply long strokes from one side all the way around to the other side (follow the shape of a dome).

4. Use small circular pressure on the upper abdominal area. Move to the other side of the table and knead the fleshy part on the side, directly under the armpits.

5. Once again, run the fingers between the rib cage cartilage, starting at the back and going around to the front to the joining point of the sternum.

6. Then move to the neck and massage by using the forefinger and middle finger to work along the neck. Also carefully and very gently press the vertebrae. Use small circular kneading motions in this area.

7. Move back to the upper torso area and tap the fingers in fast rhythmic motion along the top of the flesh. Then by placing the hand firmly over small areas, making sure that the palm is pressed against the skin, create a cupping effect. Create a vibrating effect by gently shaking the area then lifting the hand off the skin very quickly (called the "suction technique").

8. Turn the person over. Place the palm of his or her hand around the shoulder blade. Use the same long strokes to massage the rib cage cartilage. Use the same kneading motions to massage the fleshy area at the sides and to once again massage the neck area.

9. The suction technique can be used on the back.

10. End with an overall gentle rub for as long as desired.

Abdominal breathing

Abdominal breathing is widely known as the best method of breathing to relax the mind and body. It is also easier to grasp than diaphragmatic breathing. Your abdominal muscles go all the way from your pelvic bone up to your sternum and lower rib cage. These muscles tighten when you are scared or stressed. In order to breathe deeply, they need to stay relaxed. The aim of breathing training is to train the abdominal muscles to be naturally relaxed most of the time, but also to be able to tighten them and make them strong when necessary.

We will first learn abdominal breathing in a lying position. Later, you can try it when sitting. You should only use throat breathing—keep checking throughout that you are doing this. (Technically we don't breathe into the abdomen. It expands as a result of the downward movement of the diaphragm. But it's helpful to "imagine" you are breathing into the abdominal area.)

ABDOMINAL INHALATION

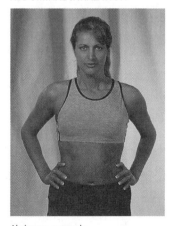

Abdomen expands.

ABDOMINAL EXHALATION

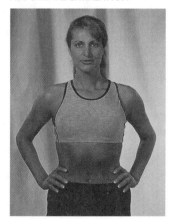

Abdomen contracts.

BASIC EXERCISE—STAGE 1

ABDOMINAL INHALATION

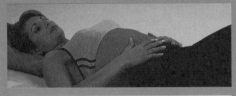

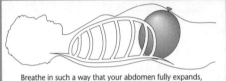

Breathe in such a way that your abdomen fully expands,
as if a balloon is inflating inside your belly.

1 Lie down and make sure you are warm and comfortable. It is better to bring your knees up, but position yourself as feels best for you. Place a towel or small pillow behind your head so that your chin is toward your chest and your neck is lengthened.

ABDOMINAL EXHALATION

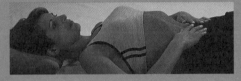

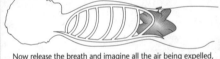

Now release the breath and imagine all the air being expelled,
like air is released from a balloon.

2 Place your hands on your abdomen with fingers pointing inward toward the belly button.

Where to place your hands during abdominal breathing

When the instructions ask you to breathe into the abdomen, place your fingertips on your belly button. Use your imagination and visualize pulling the breath only to that point, not to the upper chest as well.

3 Inhale very slowly and deeply through the nose and intentionally draw the breath to the belly button area so the abdomen expands. On a scale of 1–10, the volume of the breath is one or two, and it is as soft as possible. Begin to lengthen your inhalation and exhalation as much as you can.

4 Bring your awareness to your hands. Begin inhaling so that the abdomen expands. Go slowly. Fill up a little first, then gradually increase the amount, but still breathe gently. Use your hands to feel what is happening. If you are breathing and your upper chest is moving but you cannot feel your abdomen expanding or

decreasing, then you are breathing incorrectly. Slightly increase the pressure on your abdomen; focus, and imagine pulling the breath down to your belly button.

5 After a few minutes of proper abdominal breathing, you should find you naturally fall into a rhythmical and harmonious breathing pattern and start to feel relaxed. This indicates that you are correctly performing abdominal breathing, and you can progress to the next stage.

BASIC EXERCISE—STAGE 2

6 Start to increase the amount of breath being drawn in and expelled. Adjust the volume of breath to three on the scale, but make sure you do not begin at any point to breathe too hard (otherwise you will not be able to lengthen the breath or totally expand the abdomen). Slowly and gently increase the amount of breath in and out.

7 Move your hands to the sides so that the base of your hands is on the sides of your abdomen. Now breathe so that the sides of your abdomen also expand. Do 10 of these, making sure your hands move outward to the sides as you breathe in.

8 Increase the pressure of your hands, and this time see if you can breathe in such a way that only the sides of your abdomen increase and decrease. It helps to imagine you have an oblong balloon inflating and deflating in the middle of your belly.

9 Now take big, deep abdominal breaths and aim to expand both parts of the abdomen: front, and sides. Do this a few times and then rest.

ADVANCED EXERCISE

1 To fine-tune your abdominal breathing, lie down and place an object on your abdomen that has weight, such as a heavy book. (Make sure the object is not too heavy and does not make you feel uncomfortable.) Inhale and exhale moving the object on your abdomen without obviously moving anything else such as your chest or rib cage.

2 Repeat, but this time at the top of your inhalation, secure a measuring tape firmly around your upper chest. Breathe in and out, expanding the abdomen, moving the book only. Your chest should be up and open and should not have moved or dropped at all from your starting point, indicated by the measuring tape when you first secured it. This exercise teaches you to emphasize the abdomen when breathing. The diaphragm is incorporated naturally, and the rib cage should barely move. For this exercise, we want *only* zone 3 to be working.

Diaphragmatic breathing

As previously mentioned, diaphragmatic breathing is a much more challenging method of breathing to learn than abdominal breathing.

Your breathing can best meet the demands of a strenuous activity when the diaphragm is fully utilized. You can control the "kind" of breath you produce and adjust it according to the demand.

Furthermore, when the diaphragm and abdomen are relaxed, they can move slowly, powerfully, upward, downward and in a controlled manner.

If you want to consciously lengthen an exhalation, you need to keep the abdomen relaxed—rather than tight—even as it's moving. This allows a gradual movement upward. It is only at the end of the exhalation that you are required to consciously tighten your abdominal muscles.

Only when you can fully relax and tense the abdominal muscles and diaphragm can you inhale and exhale for a lengthened period. You need to learn to be able to relax or tighten the abdominal muscles and diaphragm at will. For the exhalation, they must be relaxed in order to move as you consciously direct them, enabling you to move them upward. If you are not relaxed, the breath will stop as soon as the abdomen and diaphragm are tightened, which will probably be after three or four seconds. However, by relaxing them, you can exhale for a lengthened period of time. The length of the inhalation is determined by your ability to keep the diaphragm initially firm, then, after a certain point, relaxed until it contracts.

You need to be able to emphasize and move the rib cage and barely move the upper chest at all times; and the abdomen only some of the time. (It is acceptable to have minimal movement of the upper chest, although experienced breathers are proficient at it without any apparent movement.) You also need to be able to move the rib cage inward and outward without dropping the ribs or upper chest.

When I ask you to work the diaphragm and rib cage area, place the heels of your hands on the rib cage on the sides of your body, not in the middle. Your hands stay positioned on that part of the body, so when you exhale and move your ribs inward, keep a good grip on the skin and allow the hands to move as the ribs do. As you exhale, the fingertips will move toward each other and finally touch at the end of the breath. As you are inhaling, the ribs should open outward back to the open position and your hands will part accordingly.

EXERCISE 1

The following exercise allows you to explore the rim of the diaphragm and rib cage. This will help you understand them more and visualize your own rib cage and diaphragm, as well as following the instructions below for using your hands to feel them. If you are pregnant or injured or have painful ribs, either use the visuals only during this exercise or very gently touch the surface of your ribs.

First, sit on a chair or cross-legged on the floor or a bed. Make sure zone 2 is as bare as possible and that your fingers are too. Start off by spending some time becoming acquainted with your rib cage. If you cannot see and feel your ribs, then dig deeper. Begin from the middle (the sternum). Then probe your fingers and feel the ribs one by one. Follow them all the way around. Notice the space between the ribs. Become aware of the whole rib cage structure and its barrel-like appearance.

PEAK POINT

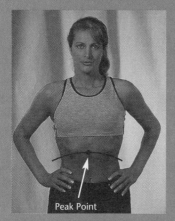
Peak Point

Sit in front of a mirror. Examine the rib cage closely. Next, find the end of your sternum and place a couple of fingers there and press your fingers in at that point—I call this the "peak point" of the diaphragm. Your diaphragm is positioned at this level, spreading like a dome or an umbrella over the abdominal contents. At this point, your fingers are feeling the "peak point"—the rim of the diaphragm—while the rest is inside the rib cage separating the lungs from your abdomen.

EXPLORING THE DIAPHRAGM

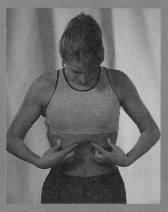

Next, place your fingers on the diaphragm area at the peak point. The forefingers are on top, and the other fingers follow downward along the diaphragm. We are now aiming to develop sensitivity to what the diaphragm actually does, and what it feels like during an inhalation and an exhalation. The more knowledge and awareness you have about how the diaphragm muscle works and what it does in different circumstances, the more chance you have of mastering it and being able to control it. Start breathing in and out using a firm throat breath. For the purposes of this particular exercise, deliberately allow your abdomen to expand more than normal when breathing in. Follow the movement of the inhalation and exhalation with your fingers. Feel the diaphragm as it moves up and down. Familiarize yourself with it and how it functions as a muscle. Breathe for a little while. Rest, then repeat.

EXERCISE 2

This time with fingers in the same position, breathe out and follow the diaphragm inward with your fingers and then pause. Keep your fingers pressed into your body as far as is comfortable. You need to keep applying a gentle pressure to make sure your fingers stay right in there. Now breathe in for two seconds. You should feel a pressure from the diaphragm against your fingertips. Even though the diaphragm wants to push downward, keep feeling the pressure of it resisting against your fingers. Repeat this several times.

EXERCISE 3

This exercise is a little complicated, but it is important in achieving a lengthy inhalation. Again, be as bare-chested as possible in front of a mirror. We are now going to continue on from the last exercise where your fingers felt the pressure of the diaphragm. Once again, position your fingers, making sure they are pressed into your body against the diaphragm as much as possible. Also place a thumb on each side in the middle of the ribs. Breathe in for two seconds, mentally directing the breath to the ribs only.

Your aim is to breathe in such a way that you do not feel any pressure against your fingers from the diaphragm until the end of the breath. If you are unable to grasp this exercise at first, keep trying until you do. Tell yourself that the body is capable of doing it, and allow your mind to work out how. Trust yourself that you can control your diaphragm exactly as you command.

If you can do it properly for the first two seconds, pause and inhale for another two seconds. Aim to do five short breaths without feeling pressure on the diaphragm (ribs only expanding). Only when you can hold the diaphragm in an upright position for a long time will you be able to breathe a lengthened breath and fully expand the sides of the ribs. You must learn how to keep the diaphragm up and breathe so the ribs expand first, rather than the upper chest or even the abdomen. You should feel no pressure from the diaphragm until the very end of your inhalation. For lengthened breathing, there should be a gradual release of the diaphragm, rather than any abrupt pressure against your fingertips.

EXERCISE 4

This is the same as exercise 3, except that you breathe in one long continuous inhalation without any pausing. You must breathe in very slowly or it will not work. Keep your throat breath very gentle and soft.

Follow the instructions as in exercise 3 in front of the mirror, placing the fingers on the diaphragm and thumbs on the side of the ribs. Begin to draw breath in slowly and bring it to the peak point. From there, imagine letting the breath begin on the first rib. As you keep inhaling, let the breath gradually spread outward toward the end of the ribs.

About halfway through the breath, you may begin to imagine very slowly releasing the diaphragm. It should be deliberately released so slowly and smoothly that you barely feel it on your fingertips. Then regulate the breath with your body movements to complete the inhalation.

Your focus should always be on expanding the ribs and at the same time preventing your diaphragm from flattening out and moving downward too quickly. *Tip: use your fingers to press each section of the ribs, thereby directing the breath to that area* (see photos on page 107). This is a necessary and helpful technique to use in the initial stages of learning.

You will find at this point that the diaphragm will automatically begin to release and move downward—it's up to you to stop it from dropping or moving too quickly or abruptly.

Do this exercise until you fully grasp it. Until you become proficient at it, you can hold the diaphragm up with your fingers for the first few seconds or more and release your fingers toward the end of the breath. Eventually, you will achieve a good inhalation the whole way through without needing to use your fingers to hold the diaphragm up. But until then, you will need all the help you can get. The purpose of holding the diaphragm with your fingers is to give you the sensation of what holding the diaphragm at the peak point feels like.

Even though it may take a bit of practice, after mastering these exercises, your inhalation will improve automatically. You will be able to control your diaphragm from start to end, instead of letting it drop rapidly from the beginning. So once you are confident with how you have progressed, try to breathe in a long inhalation without using your hands. Use the mirror to check that you are doing it correctly. You might find it helpful to *imagine* that you are using your fingers to hold the diaphragm up.

TRAINING THE DIAPHRAGM—LYING DOWN

EXPLORING THE DIAPHRAGM

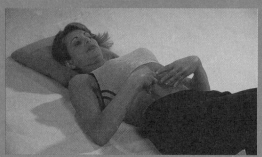

Now try all the exercises lying down. Remember all the principles about proper posture on the floor:
- chin toward the chest
- neck lengthened
- shoulders flat against the floor
- chest up and open
- tilt the pelvis (hip area) properly
- bend your knees up so that you can support your back

You must maintain all of the above for the whole duration of the exercise, otherwise you cannot achieve successful results. Because the floor is supporting you, you can focus and concentrate on the inhalation completely. Once again, use your imagination and really "feel" what is going on inside your rib cage area.

The following exercises are two of the most important in this book. So if you are really serious about improving the quality and duration of your breath, take your time and keep practicing them.

ISOLATION EXERCISE

In order to completely focus on the diaphragm and all of zone 2, you will need two books. Use a book that is reasonably weighted but not so that it is uncomfortably heavy. Place one on your abdomen on top of your belly button and the other on your upper chest (on your sternum). Constantly make sure your neck is lengthened and your chin is toward your chest. The aim is to keep the books as still as possible and move mainly the middle section—the rib cage and the diaphragm. If you keep the abdominal muscles up and held firm, you will find you will be able to move the middle section without much movement from the upper chest. It also helps to lift your chest high and keep your shoulders flat against the floor.

DIAPHRAGM EXERCISE

This is an exercise to help you vary the softness and intensity of your diaphragm. In order to do it effectively, you will need to use an imagination exercise and also adjust the volume of your breath, as you did in the throat breathing section (see pages 52–57).

Let's begin with the imagination exercise. Close your eyes and picture your hand opening as wide as possible and closing into a fist. On a scale of 1 to 10, think of 1 as your hand wide open and 10 as your fist squeezed as hard as possible. Now I want you to pretend your diaphragm is your hand and use your creative mind to allow your diaphragm to spread out and become as soft as possible. Next imagine squeezing the diaphragm as much as you can, aiming for a 10.

Now we will try it for real, although there is no reason why you can't use your imagination to work the diaphragm. I do and it works for me! If you're not sure of how to contract your diaphragm, then cough and you will feel it. Start throat breathing and vary the intensity of your breathing and also relax and contract the diaphragm. Can you relax it so it feels it is at 1 on the scale? Can you squeeze as much as possible so that it is at 10, but without allowing your shoulders or upper chest to drop forward or be too involved? You know the importance of the diaphragm by now, so this is an exercise worth practicing and mastering. I guarantee that you will be rewarded for your effort.

DIAPHRAGM EXERCISE—SITTING AND STANDING

You are learning how to control the diaphragm while you are lying down and fully supported by the floor. In order to develop the diaphragm in different ways, try the above exercise in a sitting and standing position compared to lying down. Some people actually find it easier to do in a sitting position. However, everyone finds the standing position the hardest. But I highly recommend you work your diaphragm in a standing position as well so that you can strengthen, tone and control it from a different angle. It will also give you incredible versatility with your breathing ability, especially if you have trouble with your breathing when you are exercising. It will assist you greatly when you are exercising by giving you:

- more control with your movements.
- extra strength.
- an increase in stamina and endurance.

THE PELVIC TILT

The pelvic tilt is extremely helpful for a couple of reasons. Firstly, it can help you breathe a full breath and secondly, it can make it easier for you to effectively move your abdominal muscles and diaphragm in the initial learning stages. It can also prevent your upper chest and shoulders rolling forward off the floor.

When I talk about the pelvic area, I am referring to your whole hip area. If it helps, think of it as zone 3. Tilting the pelvis during the first few moments of exhaling helps the diaphragm and abdomen move upward. Initially, you will

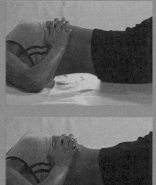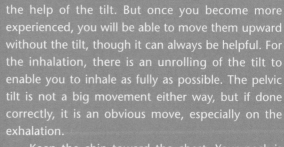 probably only be able to move them upward with the help of the tilt. But once you become more experienced, you will be able to move them upward without the tilt, though it can always be helpful. For the inhalation, there is an unrolling of the tilt to enable you to inhale as fully as possible. The pelvic tilt is not a big movement either way, but if done correctly, it is an obvious move, especially on the exhalation.

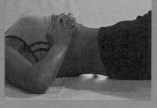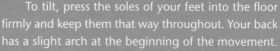 Keep the chin toward the chest. Your neck is lengthened and your shoulders are flat. Feet are pressed firmly and evenly onto the floor.

To tilt, press the soles of your feet into the floor firmly and keep them that way throughout. Your back has a slight arch at the beginning of the movement.

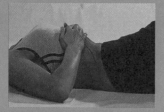 Do not lift your buttocks too far off the floor. Make sure you keep your shoulders pinned to the floor the whole time. Keep your diaphragm and abdominal areas relaxed and imagine them moving upward slowly.

With the shoulders still on the floor, the abdomen pushes the diaphragm up into the peak point and the rib cage is closed inward. Notice how at the finish, there is no longer an arch in the spine; it is rounded in the opposite direction. If you have lifted your shoulders off the floor and there is a curve in your spine, you are tightening your abdominal muscles too soon, and you have not tilted enough. Spread and "melt" the shoulders into the floor, relax the abdominal muscles and diaphragm, and tilt some more.

The pelvic tilt should be used only half the time for the inhalation and exhalation. On the exhalation, tilt until the back flattens, then stop. On the inhalation, you begin the tilt halfway through the breath (for the first half there is no tilting, only movement with the rib cage).

Overview of diaphragmatic breathing

EXHALATION

| STAGE 1 | STAGE 2 | STAGE 3 | STAGE 4 |

INHALATION

| STAGE 1 | STAGE 2 | STAGE 3 | STAGE 4 |

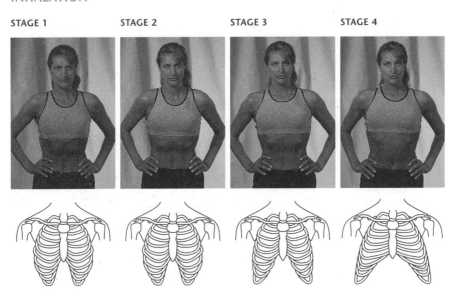

The diaphragmatic exhalation

We will now begin our first lesson for the diaphragmatic exhalation. This is much more technical than abdominal breathing, but the results are well worth the effort. At first, it may seem as if there are many points to remember, but keep practicing and you will soon put it all together.

The diaphragmatic exhalation significantly incorporates the abdomen, but another focus is the lower rib cage to the extent that you can see and feel it opening and closing. When you can perform this kind of breathing properly, you will be able to direct your breath and body to do exactly as you wish, and you can begin to fine-tune and vary the exhalation.

Before we begin, I would like to remind you to keep checking your posture at all times. Aim for the perfect posture described on pages 64–70. Also be wary of a bad habit that often occurs during the exhalation; dropping the shoulders and upper chest in an attempt to expel that extra bit of breath. The chest falls forward with the shoulders rolling off the floor, dropping downward. The chest then drops and sinks, and does not allow for a full or good quality breath. Whether this occurs at the start of the exercise or toward the end, it is incorrect procedure and should be avoided. The challenge is to complete the whole exhalation without any obvious involvement at all from zone 1.

It doesn't matter if at the beginning the exhalation is a bit shorter than you would like. The only way that you will achieve a full and lengthened exhalation is if you keep the chest and shoulders raised and still. By using zone 2 instead of the upper chest, you will ultimately achieve a much longer and better quality breath. Make it a point to always aim for quality no matter what it takes. Duration can be achieved after quality has been instilled.

In the early stages of your training, you may find it difficult to keep the shoulders and upper chest still. This is normal. As you practice, you will begin to find that you can reach halfway through the exhalation before there is any obvious upper chest movement. Eventually, you will be able to reach the end of a lengthened exhalation without any obvious movement of the shoulders or upper chest.

The other tricky part of the exhalation is in controlling the timing of the rib cage closing inward. If you close the ribs straight away, the abdomen is limited in its range of movement and the exhalation will end in a short and incomplete breath. The rib cage must remain wide open in order for the abdomen to be able to fully work its way into the ideal position for a lengthened exhalation.

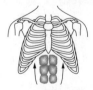 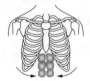

The diaphragmatic exhalation

STAGE 1

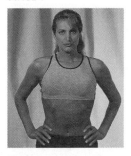 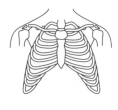

The rib cage is opened up as much as possible (remember to only use good quality throat breathing). The upper chest and shoulders are upright, and remain that way throughout.

STAGE 2

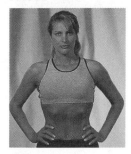 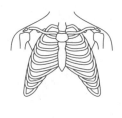

In order to achieve a lengthened exhalation, you must keep the rib cage open for as long as you can. This allows room for the abdomen to slowly and gradually move upward.

STAGE 3

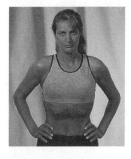 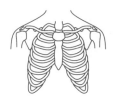

After you have drawn the abdomen upward, slowly and gradually close the rib cage inward.

STAGE 4

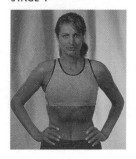 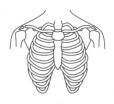

Only toward the end should you tighten the abdomen, and finish so the rib cage is closed inward as much as possible without dropping the shoulders and upper chest.

Remember: for the diaphragmatic exhalation, the emphasis and focal points are predominately the diaphragm, lower rib cage and abdomen.

PRACTICING THE EXHALATION—LYING DOWN

STAGE 1

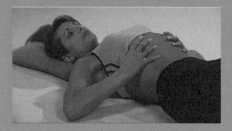

STAGE 2

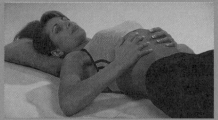

STAGE 3

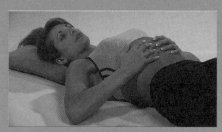

STAGE 4

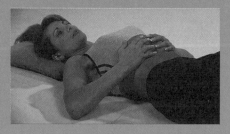

When I ask you to work the diaphragm and rib cage area, place the heels of your hands on the rib cage on the sides of your body, not in the middle. Your hands stay on that part of the body, so when you exhale and move your ribs inward, keep a good grip on the skin and allow the hands to move as the ribs do. (As you exhale, the fingertips will move toward each other, finally touching at the end of the breath. As you inhale, the ribs should open outward back to the open position.)

Your knees should be bent a little, with your pelvis relaxed and spread evenly on the floor. Your back arches naturally in this position so allow that to happen. Your shoulders are relaxed and spread out and open evenly. Lengthen and widen them so that the whole chest area is up and open (like a barrel). Your chin is pointing in the direction of your chest and your neck is lengthened. Pressing feet into the floor, move the pelvis upward. The spine will very slowly begin to flatten and should be completely flat by the end of the exhalation. The chest and rib cage are open and round at the beginning; *your aim is to keep the chest constantly upright and maintain perfect posture throughout the entire exhalation.*

If your chest or rib cage drops, it means you have not synchronized the breath, diaphragm and rib cage together. You need to work all three of them as a unit, slowly and gradually coming to a close, so that all body parts complete their individual tasks by the end of the exhalation.

The ribs should have moved inward but should not have dropped. There is still an openness even though you have exhaled completely. You must finish the exhalation without lowering the upper chest at all, or you will never achieve a fully completed deep and lengthened breath. By working the diaphragm in this manner, it is strengthened. It is only when the diaphragm is stronger that you can move on to increase the duration of your exhalation, and properly perform power breathing.

Begin by inhaling a nice deep breath. (Fill up your lungs, but not so much that you are uncomfortable and are desperate to exhale.) The fundamental aspect for this part is to have your whole rib cage and chest as up and open as possible. Your sternum should be raised upward as high as possible. Keep reminding yourself that if your chest and/or ribs have dropped at any point, you will not be able to perform the exercise properly.

Using the pelvic tilt (see page 94), breathe out and move the abdominal area upward without the rib cage or chest moving at all. Begin with tiny movements, making sure the abdomen and diaphragm are still relaxed.

Remember: if the abdomen is tightened too early, it will not fully move upward. This will result in the breath being instantly cut short. Release any urgency or tension, remain relaxed and take your time.

Constantly check to make sure you are not doing the following:

- dropping the upper chest and rib cage
- rolling the shoulders forward off the floor
- tightening the abdominal muscles throughout the movement, other than the last three to five seconds

You will need to use self-talk throughout this process. Constantly remind yourself with the helpful phrases, "I have all the time in the world to breathe in," and "My breathing is made up of small components." As you already know, it is essential that you take your time when practicing good quality breathing. And when continuously exhaling for a long time you need to remember that your breathing has to be broken up into components—that is, in your mind rather than out loud. The breath should be one smooth, continuous sound without any abruptness. Imagine that it comprises a whole stream of mini-breaths joined as one.

The ideal is not to *consciously* tighten or tense the abdomen throughout 95 percent of the movement. Only at the final stage, for about the last five seconds, do you begin to gradually tighten the abdomen. (This is one of the main reasons why proficient breathers can breathe as brilliantly as they do.) It is only in the last three seconds that you purposely tighten the abdomen as much as you can in order to complete a lengthened exhalation.

If the abdomen is tightened after the first few seconds of breathing out, you will find your exhalation will not continue for very long. This will result in a short, incomplete exhalation and will leave you frustrated because, no matter how much you try, you will not be able to breathe out for any longer.

The next important task is to detect the precise point at which you tighten the abdominal muscles. The tension that is habitually locked in must be consciously released in order to proceed. If you try too hard and attempt to force the abdomen to relax, it will never work. Simply tell yourself to let go of any tension in the abdominal area. You cannot progress on to the next step if the abdominal muscles are tense because the diaphragm will not be able to move effectively for a full deep breath. Instead, the upper chest will automatically expand.

So keep reminding yourself of the importance of keeping the abdominal area relaxed to enable it to move upward. As you master the ability to move the abdomen in a relaxed state, you will find you can lift it high up. The higher the better because this means the diaphragm is taking more time to complete its full movement, which results in a longer exhalation. Also, when the diaphragm is at peak point, it gives you excellent control. In this position you can move the rib cage exactly as you command, i.e., inward, outward, slow, fast, gently or powerfully.

You will know when the exhalation has been performed properly and reached its absolute completion when the following occur exactly at the same time:

- the sound of the exhalation has finished.
- the abdomen is tensed to what feels like its maximum.
- the upper chest is still up and open and the shoulders are flat on the floor.
- both sides of the rib cage are in toward each other as much as possible and still rounded, like a barrel.

While you might be used to seeing a dropped chest at the completion of an extended exhalation, for good quality breathing to occur, this is incorrect. Have you ever seen a singer's chest and posture collapse at the end of a note? Even the most powerful opera singers perform with their upper chest constantly up and open.

Faults to look out for during the exhalation:

- Sound and movement not finishing at the same time. The breath must finish at the exact time of the final close of the ribs and a fully tensed abdomen. (One should not have finished before the other.)
- The sound of the breath weakening at any point, especially toward the end. It must be smooth, consistent and relaxed, yet still with a certain amount of strength in it, even toward the very end.

- The breath being too short and too hard.
- Shoulders rolling forward off the floor.
- The rib cage dropping. (The ribs should move in toward each other, not downward.)

The diaphragmatic inhalation

In normal breathing, the inhalation process (in terms of airflow) is slower compared with the exhalation, even though the duration of the exhalation is longer. So for normal (abdominal) breathing, the two phases of inhalation and exhalation are not the same, with respect to airflow and duration.

Breathing training teaches you how to inhale much longer and deeper than for the normal breath. The inhalation process that you will now be instructed on is not that much different from what you have learned with the diaphragmatic exhalation. The principles are basically the same, so you will not need to learn a whole new set of unfamiliar instructions.

Almost everyone finds the inhalation the most challenging aspect to grasp— so don't feel frustrated or despondent if you don't achieve results immediately.

Let's re-cap on significant points you have covered so far for the exhalation, which are also relevant for the inhalation; you should breathe in a slow, relaxed manner, and while there should be no sign of force, the breath does need to have some "oomph."

The fundamental aspects crucial to successfully learning how to improve and lengthen the inhalation are:

- how much control you have over the breath and diaphragm.
- how slowly and gently you breathe.
- how you regulate the breath with the relevant body parts and movements involved.

Again, as with the exhalation, the biggest mistake is to inhale with an emphasis on the upper chest area. It is your mental commands to the body and a powerful use of throat breathing that will help to move the rib cage and control the diaphragm. You do not need to move your shoulders and chest. If you do, then you will lose the power, strength and control that the diaphragm can give, and also the duration and quality of breath.

You must give your mind specific directions, thoughts and visual images, otherwise you are more likely to move the upper chest. I have found certain images to be useful when practicing the inhalation, such as a bird slowly and gracefully opening its wings to represent the rib cage opening and closing. (I will give you more examples of useful images as we move through this section.)

The abdomen will move toward the end of the inhalation, but only a fraction compared with abdominal breathing. As with the exhalation in diaphragmatic breathing, the main activity is in zone 2, with only the diaphragm and rib cage area fully expanding. The abdomen will expand to some extent, but only a little, which should be toward the end of the inhalation. You should allow the abdomen to expand naturally during the inhalation, as the ribs open up. If you focus on expanding the abdomen more than on opening the rib cage out sideways, you will change the style of breath, and your inhalation will not be as long. Remember, the diaphragm is the master of breathing, so put the emphasis on it for the best results, especially for the diaphragmatic inhalation.

If you are still having difficulty moving the rib cage without obviously moving the abdomen, go back and reread the section on emphasizing body parts (see pages 61–63) and practice those exercises again.

IMAGINATION EXERCISE

I have already mentioned the importance of using your imagination during breathing training. If you want to achieve a "deep and lengthened" inhalation, it is even more important. The following imagery exercise is one I use myself, and it is what I teach during breathing training.

Begin by placing the diaphragm upright at peak point. At the same time, picture that your shoulders are going in a downward direction. They should not move at all, but we imagine that they do in order to counteract the tendency to lift the shoulders upward when inhaling.

When you are trying to breathe long and deeply, do not think of the breath being inhaled from the abdomen and moving upward toward the upper chest, but rather visualize the diaphragm as an umbrella. Imagine it is creating a seal, preventing the air from going into the abdominal area. Now I would like you to imagine that as you inhale very slowly, your breath is entering your body in the manner and direction of a glass of water when you are drinking it. Think of tiny components of breath as if they were little sips entering the diaphragm area slowly and smoothly.

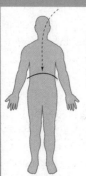

Imagine your inhalation entering your body in the direction water does when drinking. Visualize the breath stopping at the diaphragm.

Correct

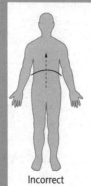

Do not think of the breath beginning from the abdomen and being inhaled in an upward direction. This approach results in the inhalation being short, abrupt, and ending up in the upper chest area, making it an upper chest breath.

Incorrect

The diaphragmatic inhalation

STAGE 1

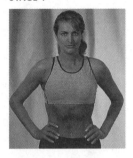
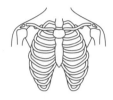

The rib cage is closed inward as much as possible. The upper chest is upright and remains that way throughout.

STAGE 2

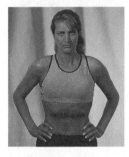
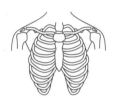

In order to achieve a lengthened inhalation, you must use a good quality throat breath to pull the breath in, and at the same time, you must continue to keep the rib cage inward (use your hands to help you, see page 107). It is really important to do this stage for as long as possible.

STAGE 3

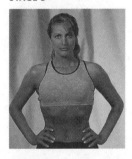
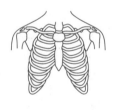

At this stage, you gradually open up the (lower) rib cage, but still aim to keep the abdomen upward and held firmly.

STAGE 4

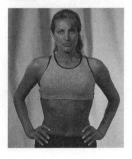
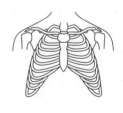

Only in the last stage toward the end of the inhalation should you (gradually) completely relax your abdomen. By the end, the rib cage has opened as much as possible, without the shoulders and upper chest lifting. The abdomen has expanded only a little bit.

PRACTICING THE INHALATION

To inhale for as long as you possibly can, you need to make sure you begin at the end of your exhalation. Both sides of the rib cage need to be drawn in together to a tight close at the end of your exhalation. You should keep the diaphragm lifted and upright, with a firm grip on it.

However, do not grip in a restrictive manner, otherwise you will not be able to breathe in smoothly and for an extended length of time. If the abdomen is tightened to its extreme as your starting point, after inhaling for a few seconds, you will soon become exhausted and you will struggle with the inhalation. So before you begin inhaling, it is really important that your abdomen is consciously tightened only so it is firm enough to be held upward, which consequently supports the diaphragm.

At the starting point of the inhalation, the diaphragm must be upright at peak point, and held firmly, yet relaxed. While we do not want it too tight, we also do not want to make the mistake of allowing the diaphragm to relax so much that it will immediately drop from the upright position when we begin inhaling. If you allow this to happen, you will lose your control and also the duration of your inhalation will be considerably shortened.

If you feel you need help in keeping the diaphragm upright initially, you may use the technique to hold the diaphragm up with your fingers.

Draw in the breath—concentrate on using throat breathing only and be very aware of pulling in the breath. *Once again, imagine you are drawing breath as if you were drinking water downward and NOT from the abdomen upward* (see diagram on page 102). Although you must remain relaxed, this is not a passive pulling in of the breath. You must draw the breath in with "gentle power" and with conscious awareness, specifically emphasizing and working the diaphragm.

When you are aiming for a long inhalation, the key is to keep the diaphragm at the peak point for as long as you can. For the first part of the inhalation, you must imagine breathing into that specific point without moving anything else, including your rib cage.

Picture a visual image of the breath being pulled in directly to the diaphragm at the peak point, in a gradual and very slow manner (the slower, the better so that there is no obvious movement). All of zone 2 is supported by the contracted and drawn up abdominal muscles. In this manner, the breath is inhaled for as long as possible.

Take your time as you slowly breathe in, and little by little expand the rib cage. If you feel an urge to try to breathe in all at once and your rib cage is opening up too quickly, remind yourself to slow down and breathe in small components. Remind yourself that you have all the time in the world. It's only by breathing gently and moving the body parts gradually that you can detect precisely when you begin to use incorrect breathing form.

When I am working one-on-one with people, I carefully watch them for any interfering habits. When I detect that something is wrong, I show them how to do it properly. Then, we progress to the next step, and so on. As you are your own instructor, the mirror and/or the feeling of your body and the duration of your breathing all will help to tell you when something is not progressing ideally—or is ideal, for that matter!

Later, when you are able to breathe slowly, you will be ready to learn how to breathe quickly and powerfully. But for now, you must learn how to breathe very slowly. You will find it really helpful to keep reminding yourself to "go slowly."

Check yourself after you have completed your full inhalation to make sure that the ribs have opened outward. Have the shoulders been raised? If they have, at what point did they begin to move upward? (Gently relax them back into their proper position.) Does your upper chest seem fuller? Exactly when did this happen? Did it happen a little or a lot? Can you repeat the exercise, expanding the rib cage with almost no movement from the upper chest or even the abdominal muscles?

During the next stage, the rib cage opens up. This happens really s-l-o-w-l-y and in small components. If you move or drop your rib cage abruptly, it will cause your diaphragm to drop from the upright position. This will result in the abdominal area automatically expanding, making it an abdominal rather than a diaphragmatic breath.

After you have drawn in the breath for a while, the rib cage will be ready to open up. Slowly proceed, but don't let the diaphragm drop. It will disrupt the synchronicity, flow and length of the inhalation. As the breath continues, the diaphragm will slowly but surely begin to flatten out somewhat. The longer and deeper the breath, the more the lungs will be filled and ventilated.

By the time you have completed three quarters of the exhalation, the abdominal area will begin to expand, but only a little. *By the end of the inhalation, the abdominal expansion should be only about a third of that which you experienced during abdominal breathing.* Remember, this is a specific style of breathing, so the emphasis on what expands and decreases will differ accordingly.

IMAGINE

1 Technically, the ribs go up and out. However, in order to do this particular breathing technique properly, it is really helpful at this stage of the inhalation to think of the ribs opening with two arrows in the sides of your rib cage going outward, rather than coming upward. Aim for zone 2 to be predominately working, with just a slight movement of the abdomen.

2 Use your imagination and mentally create a visual image of your ribs moving like an accordion. Your aim is to try to mimic the movement with your ribs, but barely move the upper chest and shoulders. (It definitely can be done!)

3 Another effective image is that of an oblong balloon positioned in the middle of the rib cage in zone 2, not near the upper chest or abdominal area. Imagine how the ribs would move if they surrounded this oblong-shaped balloon as it inflated and deflated.

If you concentrate on using your throat breathing effectively, you will notice that you can move your rib cage by the power of your breath. You will find that with the proper support from the abdomen, you can slowly but surely keep opening and expanding the ribs more and more. Your lungs are elastic and can be stretched to cover a tennis court, so except for the constraints of the rib cage, do not doubt their ability to hold a voluminous amount of air!

I will restate here the importance of breathing in increments. Very slowly, breathe in one tiny fraction of a breath at a time. Visualize your rib cage slowly but surely expanding horizontally one millimeter at a time. Keep the diaphragm upright and do not allow it to drop at any stage. You need to let the diaphragm gradually flatten, maintaining control until the very end of the inhalation.

You have completed a good quality and lengthened inhalation when:

- the diaphragm has flattened.
- the ribs have expanded sideways as far as possible.
- the sound of the breath finishes at exactly the same time as the ribs stop moving.
- the abdomen has expanded only a little.
- the chin is toward the chest and the neck is lengthened.
- the shoulders, upper chest and rib cage have not lifted upward.

BASIC EXERCISE

Once you learn how to improve your breathing, I recommend that you spend as much time as possible simply breathing in and out in a long, slow, deep and rhythmical manner. The first goal is to improve the quality of your breath before you try to do anything else, such as strengthen it.

STAGE 1

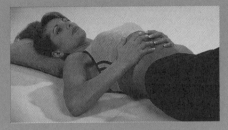

STAGE 2

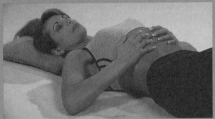

STAGE 3

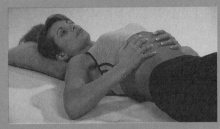

STAGE 4

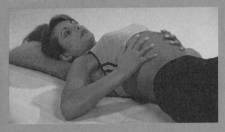

Do this exercise lying down at first. Make sure you feel comfortable and are not constricted or cold. Check that your neck is lengthened and your rib cage open. Start breathing in and out with a gentle throat breath. Try to make each breath as smooth as possible. See if you can slightly increase the length of the breath without any struggle. Simply fill up with air and release.

STAGE 1

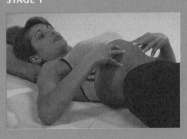

STAGE 2

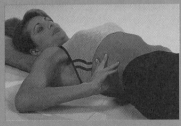

Using your fingertips is another effective way of focusing attention to the specific area you want to expand.

When you begin to feel relaxed, start to become aware of whether or not there is a difference between the inhalation and the exhalation. You will probably find that it is your exhalation that is better in quality and duration. Use this awareness exercise to learn more about the differences between the breaths and develop the weaker part/s of your breath.

Now change the breath slightly by adjusting the volume of your throat breathing. Always aim for smoothness, whether you are breathing softly or powerfully. Maintain the smoothness, but this time try to make your inhalation and exhalation slightly stronger.

ADVANCED EXERCISE

After practicing the basic exercise lying down, try doing it while sitting up. Be aware of how it feels not to have the floor supporting you. Make sure you do not allow your posture to collapse; mentally keep an eye on it. When you feel you can do the exercise reasonably well while sitting, try the most difficult position, standing.

FINE-TUNING EXERCISE FOR MOVING THE RIBS

After you have mastered small movements of the ribs inward and outward, you can begin to very slowly increase the size of the moves. Imagine that your rib cage is like an accordion or a set of bellows. With control, try to move your rib cage inward and outward, but with the following points in mind:
• The inhalation and exhalation movements are equal.
• The upper chest or rib cage does not drop at all.
• There is a sideways motion, rather than upward and downward.
• The abdomen hardly moves.

The ribs can be moved without dropping them. Try moving the rib cage so that it looks round and open, resembling the shape of a barrel, rather than looking deflated or collapsed. You need to use the diaphragm in a specific way to achieve this. Let the diaphragm control the movement and lead the way rather than the muscles of your chest. Aim to open and close the rib cage as far as possible each way, without using any incorrect breathing habits. See if you can maintain correct form the whole time, trying to elongate and use the best quality breath that you can manage.

The mega breath

I once met a Greek man whose surname was "Megas." He told me it comes from a Greek word meaning "great" as in "Alexander the Great." It was the perfect name for the following technique. This technique is similar to the breathing awareness exercises, but a lot more dynamic. The aim of the mega breath is to try to breathe your greatest, longest, biggest and best quality breath. In a sense, the mega breath is bringing together the entire breathing training program outlined in this book. It is the breath that breathes all breaths!

Practicing this technique is crucial for building all the muscles associated with powerful and lengthened breathing. Every time you practice this exercise, you strengthen the muscles that you need to breathe optimally.

In order to do the mega breath properly, you must keep in mind the following factors:

- Use only a very gentle throat breath.
- Avoid straining your face and neck—keep them relaxed.
- The shoulders must never move upward, downward, forward or backward—keep them absolutely still.
- The upper chest must not noticeably move and it should not look like it inflates on the inhale, nor deflates on the exhale—keep it in the upright position at all times so you have perfect posture.
- Challenge yourself, but be very careful! Don't strain!

Be careful not to overdo this breathing exercise. People with a competitive nature may try to push themselves beyond their limit, but you will only do more harm than good. Years of consistent training cannot be rushed in a few sessions.

It is imperative to be relaxed before you do this exercise. Always stretch the whole chest area, and take a few gentle breaths first to warm up your lungs. Also prepare yourself mentally.

I will give you instructions on the inhalation and exhalation separately. Later, you may try a mega inhalation and exhalation as one. But you must practice them in isolation first to build a foundation.

MEGA INHALATION EXERCISE

What you particularly need to watch with the inhalation is that you emphasize the diaphragm and not the upper chest. You must work only with the lower half of the rib cage and diaphragm. At no time should the upper chest (zone 1) be involved. Even the abdominal area (zone 3) should not be consciously worked. If it is noticeably moving, this will limit the ability to work zone 2 to its optimum.

If you like, you may try working both zones 2 and 3 only as a variation. But it is important to master emphasizing zone 2 by itself. Totally focusing on zone 2 specifically works the diaphragm in a way that is not typically used.

The basic principles for doing a mega inhalation are the same as for a standard diaphragmatic inhalation. You can never expand your ribs fully if you let the diaphragm immediately drop. Another very important point is that you must work in increments with your breath and body. Breathe in only a little, and move the ribs only a little at a time. You must work both the breath and movement of the rib cage together at all times, and keep the breath and movements smooth at all times. Imagine in your mind that you have all the time in the world to breathe in!

MEGA EXHALATION EXERCISE

The key is to breathe out slowly, smoothly and gradually. Think of each part of the movement as only part of a millimeter. Don't be in a rush to close the rib cage. Give yourself plenty of time to bring the abdomen and diaphragm up into zone 2. When the diaphragm is working its way toward the peak point, concentrate on taking your time to bring the rib cage inward. Also, it is crucial for you to focus your awareness on making sure no part of your body drops: not your shoulders, upper chest and particularly not your rib cage. Don't compensate for good technique by trying to force the last bit of air out by hunching your shoulders over. Constantly be aware of maintaining a proper posture, and work only the diaphragm and ribs to eliminate as much air as possible. Imagine you are breathing the air out as if you were squeezing the last bit of toothpaste out of a tube.

As you become more proficient at this, you will start to feel your diaphragm really strengthening. It's a great feeling to be able to control something so powerful and significant. And it's something you probably didn't even know you could control, let alone strengthen! You will see and feel many changes as you keep practicing the mega breath. If you exercise, you will really notice the difference. Your stamina and strength will greatly improve, and physical exertion will become effortless.

I suggest that now is a good time to reassess and time your breathing as you did on pages 46 and 50.

Breathing awareness exercises

The importance of breathing training and breathing exercises

The purpose of breathing exercises is to develop your breathing internally; they are referred to as "internal breathing exercises." While some of them can be performed with (limb or body) movements, most of them are done without any demanding movement; therefore, they do not exhaust the body in any way. While they cannot replace general exercise, ("external breathing exercises"), they can offer another dimension to your overall breathing training. Don't underestimate their power to improve your breathing and strengthen the diaphragm. Any good singer will tell you of the importance of breathing exercises as part of the training regime.

Everybody can benefit from doing different kinds of breathing exercises—both internal and external. The main aim is to practice a variety. For example, long and slow relaxation breathing is just as necessary as is vigorous breathing as a result of sports. The combination will give you a perfect balance, and it is ideal to try to incorporate both as part of your training. For your general health, it is crucial to deepen your breathing somehow. You will all choose different methods that suit you. After a while, you will start to notice a difference. You will begin to experience deep and satisfying breaths without any strain. This is a sign that you are progressing perfectly with your whole manner of breathing.

When you exhale and expel as much as you can, you will be eliminating large amounts of air. Naturally, because a vacuum has been created, your body will automatically and instinctively replace that air, driving you to much deeper inhalations than normal. So you will be giving your body an opportunity to pull in a large amount of fresh air and remove stale air.

If you are immobile because of illness or injury or you are recovering from surgery and have to bed rest, you will obviously be unable to do most forms of external breathing exercises. But you can still do internal breathing exercises while you are sitting still or lying down. And as an alternative to exercise, you can also do a separate training program where you can do some deep breathing and, at the same time, actively move your arms and/or legs.

And how about those of you who can exercise but don't because you loathe it or find it too difficult? Perhaps you may change your mind when you improve your breathing and also learn how to breathe efficiently for your chosen activity. Either way, you can also follow the suggestions for people who are immobile. As previously mentioned, it is really important (for everyone) to participate in some kind of movement or training that will deepen your breathing.

These breathing exercises develop your internal breathing in a very different way. Choose a time when you will not be disturbed. However, if you are really short of time, you can practice your breathing exercises throughout the day. For example:

• when driving (very popular)

• in traffic hold-ups

• during television commercial breaks

• while waiting in lines (inaudibly of course!)

If possible, try to have at least one proper, undisturbed practice session a week—even if for only 10 or 20 minutes—or daily for 5 minutes when you wake up and 5 minutes before you sleep.

Most of the following exercises originate from yoga. The first one is a basic exercise that will lay the foundation for the others. To time yourself, use a metronome on a beat of approximately 55 or mentally count slowly: "one . . . and . . . two . . . and . . . three . . ." etc.

Please do not strain when doing these exercises. If at any time you want to breathe normally, do so. Go back to gentle deep breathing until you feel comfortable. Do not be competitive. Master the basics thoroughly before moving on.

FOUR STAGE BREATHING

Steps 1 to 4 are considered one cycle. Do five cycles in a row.
1. INHALE . . . for a count of 4 (make sure you have fully inhaled by 4)
2. PAUSE . . . for a count of 2 (be relaxed)
3. EXHALE . . . for a count of 6 (try to be completely exhaled by 6)
4. PAUSE . . . for a count of 2 (be relaxed)

You can also try:
A. INHALE . . . 3 PAUSE . . . 3 EXHALE . . . 3 x 5 *continuously*
B. INHALE . . . 6 PAUSE . . . 3 EXHALE . . . 6 x 5 *continuously*

Begin by doing five cycles and build a solid foundation from there. It is a big mistake to progress too quickly.

SCALE BREATHING

Part A is the traditional yoga exercise, and part B is a modified version that I have created to develop the inhalation because for most people, it is the element of breathing they need to practice most.

Part A

The inhalation is half the length of the exhalation. There is no pausing with this one. (Aim to fully inhale and exhale with each breath.) Breathe in for a count of 2 and out for a count of 4, and then gradually go up the scale (breathing in for 4 and out for 8, etc.):

/ 2 / / / 4
/ / 3 / / / / / 6
/ / / 4 / / / / / / / 8
/ / / / 5 / / / / / / / / / 10
/ / / / / 6 / / / / / / / / / / / 12, etc.

Only go as high up the scale as you can without straining. Whatever number you can comfortably reach, repeat that last number, then go backward down the scale, for example 6/12, 5/10, 4/8, 3/6 and finally inhale for 2 and exhale for 4. Later, as your breathing capacity increases, you can drop the lower numbers and start a bit higher up the scale.

Part B

This exercise is the exact opposite of part A, in that you inhale for twice as long as you exhale. Breathe in for a count of 4 and out for a count of 2, and so on:

/ / / 4 / 2
/ / / / / 6 / / 3
/ / / / / / / 8 / / / 4
/ / / / / / / / / 10 / / / / 5
/ / / / / / / / / / / 12 / / / / / 6 and so on
(inhale) ——————▶ | (exhale) ——————▶ |

Remember to repeat the last number, then return to your first one.

It is normal to find part B more difficult, so take your time and do not try to go beyond your capacity. Just do the best you can.

Regulating the breath

Remember to regulate your breathing by:

* throat breathing slowly and gently.
* reducing the initial amount of air inhaled or expelled.
* controlling the use of the diaphragm.

The following exercises will help you to control and regulate your breath. Their purpose is to help you pull the breath in slowly and continuously as if you are breathing through a straw, rather than in one go as you would when blowing up a balloon. They are also good preparation exercises for sports, singing and any activity that requires regulation of the breath.

THROUGH THE STRAW

You may remember doing this one as a child. You will need a drinking straw. The aim is to breathe through the straw, not the nose. Pinch your nose if it helps to keep it sealed. We will work on the exhalation first. Breathe out through the straw as long, slow and smooth as possible without moving or dropping your upper chest. Try it a few times, then have a rest. Next, try the inhalation. You will find you cannot inhale for as long. If you breathe too much, too forcefully or too fast, the exercise will not work and you will probably end up feeling dizzy, much as you did when you were a child!   .

THROUGH THE TEETH

We will begin with the exhalation. First, relax your mouth. Inhale deeply, allowing the abdomen to expand, then bring your teeth comfortably together so that they are just touching. Gently exhale and try to breathe out for as long and as slowly as possible. Aim for 5 on the volume scale. You should make a hissing sound. Feel your belly button go inward toward your spine as you breathe out.

With the exhalation, soften the breath. Do not push too hard, or you will quickly become breathless. Repeat a few times, trying to lengthen the duration of the breath each time.

Prepare for the inhalation by exhaling deeply. Next, join your teeth together. Gently inhale (expanding your abdomen) as slow and for as long as possible, making a hissing sound. With the inhalation, concentrate on making sure the breath does not sound too weak and has some strength and power. On the volume scale, aim for about 5. Can you breathe without the breath going into the upper chest? Repeat as many times as you need to. Even if you find it difficult at first, you will soon grasp it and be able to greatly extend the duration.

During both of these exercises, can you:

- fully breathe without your upper chest, shoulders or rib cage dropping or lifting?
- breathe so that either your rib cage, abdomen or both move inward and outward?

THE COOLING BREATH

The sensation is like you are sucking in cool air. Place your tongue so it rests gently on the inside of the bottom lip. Form a circle with your mouth and slowly and softly inhale for as long as you possibly can, making sure the abdomen expands. Regulate your breath so that it is consistent and not one big gulp. As a variation, try it with an exhalation. Make sure you do not drop your chest, but rather move your belly button inward as you exhale.

Power breathing

These next two exercises help to increase the power and strength of the muscles used for breathing, especially the diaphragm.

THE BELLY BREATH

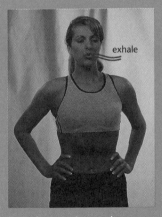
exhale

This is an excellent technique to get your circulation going, giving you a rosy glow and clearing the cobwebs from your brain. Sitting down, lying or standing, make sure your spine is straight and not hunched over, place your fingertips on your belly button. Begin by blowing out a breath as if you were blowing out hundreds of candles in one go. The exhalation should be very quick and powerful. Make sure your belly button goes in toward your spine as you breathe out. Do not be concerned about your inhalation, which will take place automatically. Just keep exhaling short, sharp, powerful breaths continuously.

Do only five gentle exhalations to start with, otherwise you may feel dizzy or light-headed. Immediately stop if this happens. It means you are doing too much, too soon. Only do a few breaths to start with and gradually add a few at a time. Aim to eventually do 10 powerful exhalations without stopping, or feeling dizzy, and build from there. This is best performed kneeling or sitting. If you can't sit, then try it standing. The belly breath is the perfect preparation for the power breath.

THE POWER BREATH

EXHALATION

INHALATION

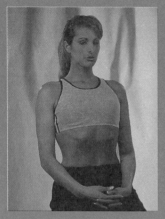

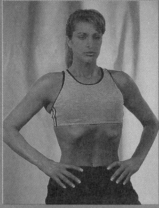

Note: You can place your hands in the position most comfortable for you.

This is an advanced version of the belly breath, and is the ultimate in challenging your ability to breathe powerfully. It is one of my favorite exercises and even the fittest athletes agree that it is the most difficult breathing exercise to perform properly. It is the most powerful and dynamic breathing exercise you will ever do. The movement is basically like a pumping motion of the diaphragm. It is the best one to use if you need to feel alert—such as before or during sports, while studying, when trying to stay awake, etc.

The power breath consists of short, sharp, powerful breaths. It can only be performed properly if you hold your upper chest and abdominal muscles upward and keep them there firmly (be careful to remain relaxed though) for the duration of the exercise. This allows the ribs to move in and out dynamically like mighty bellows! It also prevents the upper chest from dropping. The intensity of the throat breath is very strong and firm. Try it with your mouth open first. The inhalation is as active and powerful as the exhalation. Then try power breathing in and out of the nose only, with the mouth closed.

The biggest mistake I observe when people perform this technique is that they use the shoulders and upper chest to pump the breath in and out of the body—especially when trying to increase strength and power. It is really helpful to use a mirror to check yourself and make sure you are not doing this. In order to prevent the inappropriate muscles' working, remind yourself of the following important factors:

- Constantly keep your posture tall and upright.
- Concentrate on the diaphragm and rib cage area only.
- Do only very little movements with the ribs to begin with, and gradually build up from that.

The belly breath and the power breath:

- give you instant feeling of alertness.
- can help to overcome pain in certain circumstances.
- help to strengthen the diaphragm and abdomen, as well as overall quality of breathing.

VARIATIONS

As previously mentioned, in order to become truly proficient and versatile with your breathing, you should practice as many different types of breathing as possible. This will enable you to consciously and effectively change your breathing according to any demand. By now you should be aware of the different types of breathing you can achieve simply by changing the volume and pace of your breath, as discussed in the throat breathing section (see pages 52–57).

Now I would like to describe different approaches to breathing and show you how to create different effects by specifically concentrating on *how* you breathe and *which part* of the body you breathe to.

Group A: Where you can aim to breathe
1. Upper chest
2. Diaphragm
3. Abdomen (use your imagination)
4. Upper chest and diaphragm
5. Diaphragm and abdomen
6. 1, 2 and 3 altogether

Group B: How you can breathe
1. Gentle and short
2. Gentle and in-between (i.e., short and lengthy)
3. Gentle and lengthy
4. Medium and short
5. Medium and in-between (i.e., short and lengthy)
6. Medium and lengthy
7. Powerful and short
8. Powerful and in-between (i.e., short and lengthy)
9. Powerful and lengthy

You have practiced each of these separately and now we will put them together to produce a whole range of variations. In order to combine them effectively, the two crucial factors to remember are:
1. Use throat breathing.

2. Emphasize the three main areas separately—upper chest, diaphragm and abdomen.

Practice a whole range of variations by choosing one from Group A and one from Group B. I suggest you start from Group A and go through each in Group B.

You cannot apply one kind of breath to everything you do, and as you can see from this exercise, there are endless variations. I suggest that from time to time, you spend a whole session on different types of breathing so you can gain all the benefits. If, for example, you breathe only weakly and quickly mainly using the upper chest most of the time, you not only run the risk of health problems, but you will also miss the benefits that relaxation and power breathing can produce. Or if you do only abdominal breathing, you will miss out on achieving the benefits and versatility of diaphragmatic breathing.

SOUND EXERCISES

Singers use certain sounds as part of their breathing training. With this exercise, the aim is to pronounce the letter and attempt to say it for as long as possible. First, take a deep abdominal breath, then say the letter and at the same time move your belly button inward toward the spine slowly for as long as you possibly can.

AAAAAAAAAAAAAAAAAAAAAAAAAAAAAAAAAAAAAAAAAAAAAAA
EEEEEEEEEEEEEEEEEEEEEEEEEEEEEEEEEEEEEEEEEEEEEEEEEEEEEEEEE
FFFFFFFFFFFFFFFFFFFFFFFFFFFFFFFFFFFFFFFFFFFFFFFFFFFFFFFFFF
HHHHHHHHHHHHHHHHHHHHHHHHHHHHHHHHHHHHHHHHHHHH
LLLLLLLLLLLLLLLLLLLLLLLLLLLLLLLLLLLLLLLLLLLLLLLLLLLL
MMMMMMMMMMMMMMMMMMMMMMMMMMMMMMMMMMMMMMMM
NNNNNNNNNNNNNNNNNNNNNNNNNNNNNNNNNNNNNNNN
OOOOOOOOOOOOOOOOOOOOOOOOOOOOOOOOOOOOOOOOOOOOO
RRRRRRRRRRRRRRRRRRRRRRRRRRRRRRRRRRRRRR
SSSSSSSSSSSSSSSSSSSSSSSSSSSSSSSSSSSSSSSSSSSSSS
VVVVVVVVVVVVVVVVVVVVVVVVVVVVVVVVVVVVVV
ZZZZZZZZZZZZZZZZZZZZZZZZZZZZZZZZZZZZZZZZZZZZZZZZ

S and H are the two best letters to practice. Make sure you extend the actual letter and not another part. For example, F not EF, M not EM, S not ES, V not VEE.

READING EXERCISES

An excellent technique that actors use, this involves simply reading any material for as long as you can on one exhalation. The aim is to keep increasing the amount you can read before running out of a single breath.

WHISTLING

Any kind of whistling is an excellent exercise for toning the diaphragm and increasing your breathing.

COUNTING

Count out loud starting from one and keep counting until you finish your exhalation. Make a note of the number you reach and try to count past it next time.

Creating your own breathing program

There are two reasons to develop your breathing: one, for basic good health and the upkeep of a strong, healthy respiratory system; and two, for specific activities, such as sports or singing. Even if you already do some form of breathing training, the "specialized" techniques outlined in this book help you to develop your breathing ability from another angle.

Internal breathing

As mentioned in the previous chapter, I have defined two methods of breathing training: "internal" and "external." The first involves consciously working with your breathing, and there are a number of methods that develop your internal breathing in different ways. The techniques described in this book could be termed "internal." Following are some other forms of internal breathing training that have proven to be effective.

Meditation and relaxation

This is one of the best ways to improve your breathing. Both practices slow breathing down and deepen it. Every person with experience in meditation showed good quality breathing before receiving any instruction from me—more so than any other group, including those who practiced other forms of breathing training.

Yoga

The yoga breath (see pages 35–36) specifically teaches you how to breathe slowly and very deeply. There are also many other excellent breathing exercises that are taught as part of yoga. In addition, yoga teaches you to coordinate the breath with movement. (Iyengar Yoga teaches excellent diaphragmatic breathing. It is a strenuous form of yoga, so be sure to find a good instructor who will cater to your individual needs.)

Singing

Singing practice teaches excellent breath control and lengthens the duration of the breath—mainly for the exhalation. It strengthens the diaphragm and greatly increases your lung capacity.

Playing wind instruments

Musicians who play wind instruments usually exhibit a well controlled and regulated exhalation, similar to singers.

Bodywork

Some forms of bodywork such as Feldenkrais and Pilates as well as the Alexander Technique, consciously work with the breath and produce remarkable results.

T'ai chi

The breath is very slow, smooth, deep and well regulated. This is one of the most ancient and best quality forms of breathing training originating in China thousands of years ago. Even today, a large number of Chinese still practice breathing exercises (Chi Kung) daily.

Martial arts

Martial arts provide good varied training for the breath—including both gentle and powerful breathing. Martial artists use abdominal/diaphragmatic breathing. They incorporate a very powerful use of the diaphragm, which is greatly strengthened through kei, the sharp screams used when striking and kicking.

Scuba diving

Divers generally have an excellent ability to regulate the breath. They also display a good quality exhalation that is deep and slow, while the inhalation is usually reasonably well developed.

It is not easy to find a form of breathing training that works on balancing the breath so that the inhalation is developed as much as the exhalation. However, meditation, yoga, t'ai chi, diving, some aspects of martial arts, Feldenkrais and Pilates are particularly good in this area.

External breathing

Aerobic exercise is a necessary and efficient way to develop the respiratory system. It increases your lung capacity and gives your whole respiratory system a good toning. However, it does not necessarily teach good quality breathing or fix any improper breathing habits. So you may need to do specific breathing training to correct bad habits if you have any.

To get your heart rate up and increase your respiration, you need to move continuously. You could try any of the following:

- fast walking
- jogging/running
- swimming

- rowing
- cycling
- aerobics
- snow skiing
- roller-skating/blading

The exercise needs to be continuous, rather than stopping and starting. Many sports are a combination of aerobic exercise (that gets the heart rate going) and anaerobic exercise (involving bursts of intense activity) with moments when there is hardly any movement as is the case with certain sports such as tennis and football. While these sports are excellent for the respiratory system, they should be counted as additional training to your basic aerobic program. Even professional athletes of an anaerobic activity will do some form of continual aerobic exercise as part of their training.

Creating your own program

I suggest you create a basic breathing training program that suits your lifestyle in order to stay healthy. Depending on your goals and the time you have available, the program can be tailored to suit your needs. If you have time for only a limited program each week, then perhaps you can incorporate a more thorough training session once a week.

Consider the following questions to help you work out what kind of personalized program you need.

Do you need to:

- strengthen the muscles required for quality breathing?
  If so, some of them or all of them?
- increase your overall breathing capacity?
- do extra work on your inhalation/exhalation?
- improve your breathing for a specific need?
- train your breathing muscles to be more relaxed and flexible?

Choose which external/internal forms of exercise suit you. You can choose as many as you like, but you should pick at least one from each group. Spend some time considering what your specific needs are. For example, if you are a smoker or live in a polluted environment, then I suggest you constantly practice "belly breaths" and exercise early in the morning or late at night. If your inhalation is weaker than your exhalation, then you might like to work on developing it until it is similar in strength and duration to your exhalation.

All forms of good quality breathing training will improve the way you breathe. But the most effective approach is to do at least one session each week of external and internal training. If singing, t'ai chi or yoga do not appeal to you, then at least do some breathing exercises like the mega and power breaths. If aerobics or running do not appeal, then you can walk. Weight training and power sports are excellent for strengthening your breathing and developing your power breathing. For optimum results do at least a little of both internal and external breathing each week. You should also incorporate a variety of exercises, sports and breathing exercises in order to develop your breathing gently and powerfully.

Basic program

1. Daily:
   three deep abdominal breaths every morning and night. Perform the flexibility exercises, in particular the horizontal and vertical stretches.
2. 2–3 per week:
   an aerobic activity such as walking, jogging, running, cycling, aerobics, etc., for a minimum of 20–30 minutes
3. 1 per week:
   a) three mega breaths (see page 108) for inhalation and exhalation
   b) spend a few minutes breathing in front of the mirror to see if you can detect any faults—if necessary, spend 5 to 10 minutes on correcting form
   c) ten minutes of internal breathing exercises

Basic program—extra training session

If you have a very simple program and you would like to do extra activities occasionally, then it would be helpful to create an extra program. You can be flexible with time and activities chosen. For example, you can try:

* 20–30 minutes of internal breathing training exercises
* a new aerobic activity for 15 minutes, or occasionally add 15 minutes more to your current aerobic activity

When choosing the extra training session, if you have been sedentary, check with your doctor first. Listen to your body and be aware of your breathing and recovery. If you are breathless after minimal exertion, then you are pushing yourself too hard. Be sensible. If you are used to walking for 30 minutes, then build up to a 45-minute walk. And if walking is your only form of exercise, then don't attempt something too strenuous, such as a 45-minute jog. Simply increase the length or speed of an activity that you are already performing regularly or slowly introduce a new activity.

Intermediate program

This is for people who want to substantially improve their breathing. Even if you do not do anything strenuous, you can still do this program. Remember, brisk walking is an acceptable and effective form of external breathing training.

1. Daily:
   three abdominal and three diaphragmatic breaths every morning and night.
   Perform the flexibility exercises in particular the horizontal and vertical stretches.
2. 3–4 per week:
   an aerobic activity for a minimum of 30–45 minutes
3. 1 per week:
   a) five mega breaths each, for inhalation and exhalation
   b) time your longest inhalation and exhalation
   c) twenty minutes of internal breathing exercises, including the power breath
   d) a few minutes breathing in front of the mirror to see if you can detect any faults—if necessary, spend 5 to 10 minutes on correcting form.

If you do 30 minutes of aerobic activity, then eventually aim to gradually increase the intensity and/or duration as your fitness levels improve. It is crucial to create a foundation, and slowly build up your training program as you become fitter. If you progress too quickly, you will fail to develop your breathing in a healthy way, and you risk injury.

Optimum training program

This is for people whose life or livelihood literally depends on good quality breathing, such as those with respiratory problems (who have been given permission by their medical specialist), singers, athletes, etc. It is also for anyone who has the desire and the time to improve breathing to optimum levels.

1. Daily—*choose only what you are capable of*:
   a) five abdominal and five diaphragmatic breaths every morning and night. Perform the flexibility exercises, in particular the horizontal and vertical stretches, holding them for a minute each;
   b) five minutes of breathing exercises and
2. 4–6 per week:
   an aerobic activity for 30 minutes or more if you already do so
3. 1 per week:
   a) do ten mega breaths
   b) time your longest inhalation and exhalation
   c) spend a few minutes breathing in front of a mirror to see if you can detect any faults
   d) spend 10 or more minutes on correcting faults and improve on something, e.g., practice diaphragmatic breathing with no exaggerated movement from the upper chest.
4. 2–3 per week:
   30 minutes of internal breathing exercises including power breathing

How often you do the internal breathing exercises is up to you. If it really is important, or if you struggle just to breathe normally, you can do 15 minutes twice a day, every day. Or if you are an athlete and you have an injury, you can still practice your internal breathing exercises until you can train again.

Breathing training for singers and musicians

As I have mentioned, I found singers and musicians who play wind instruments to have good quality breathing. They have a long, slow, controlled and smooth exhalation and excellent control of the diaphragm.

However the ideal is to develop both the inhalation and exhalation evenly. What do your timings say? If you find that your exhalation is much better than your inhalation, I strongly suggest you do some extra work on developing the inhalation.

When both the inhalation and exhalation have greatly improved, some singers have informed me that their singing has noticeably improved. They are able to increase their control with their breathing and found that:

- their pitch became deeper and more resonant.

- they strained less and were more able to breathe easily.

- the inhalation became easier, and they could inhale a bigger breath.

- they could sing for longer with less pausing or gasping for breath.

- they could thoroughly warm up their respiratory muscles and stretch their lungs before performing.

- they had increased flexibility and strength with the diaphragm.

Also, after specific breathing training, the elasticity of the whole lung area and rib cage naturally increases and has much more flexibility. This allows for easier expansion without any restrictions. If you can breathe only into the upper chest, aim to bring the breath directly down to the diaphragm and lower rib cage area, which has an incredible ability to expand. The upper chest, however, is restricted in its ability to expand in comparison and has limitations because it is one portion of the lungs. Also, the upper chest has a narrow range of movement and cannot give you the ability to fully use the diaphragm.

I have also found that musicians who play wind instruments, such as the clarinet and trumpet, have particularly good quality and lengthy exhalations, similar to that of singers. These musicians would benefit from developing their inhalation in the same way that singers would benefit.

BREATHING FOR SPECIFIC RESULTS

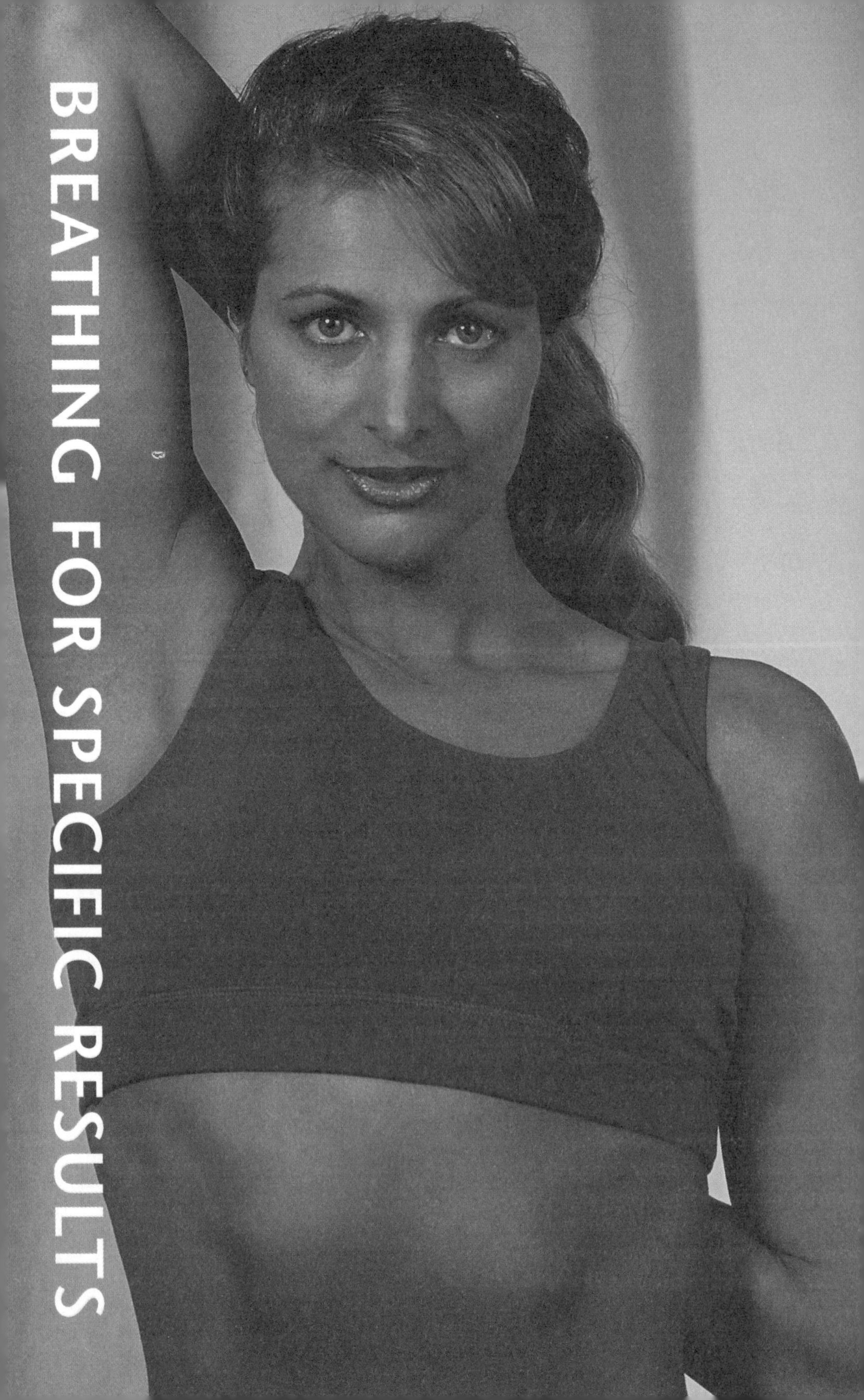

Breathing for sports and movement

I continually receive complaints from people about feeling tired and breathless during physical exertion. They come to me to learn how they can exercise without struggling and feeling so exhausted. Some people tell me their bodies give out first; others feel it is their breath. So why do many of us experience this fatigue and also become breathless so easily during physical exertion? Physiologists explain that there are a number of reasons, but the main one is that our legs fail us first. Then if the activity becomes too vigorous, we may run short of breath.

When sitting or resting, we all breathe quietly and slowly; when we become active, our breathing is programmed to become quicker, deeper and more frequent than our quiet breathing. Having worked closely with both super-fit athletes and unfit people, I have observed an obvious difference between the two groups. When fit and well-trained athletes begin exercising, they will—consciously or unconsciously— *appropriately* adjust the depth of breath to match the demand of their movements and the breath frequency required. This is one of the reasons why their performance is executed with ease.

However, if a person becomes breathless easily, there are a number of reasons why. In regards to their breathing, I have noticed quite a few differences between unfit and fit people. First, unfit people typically do not appropriately change the depth of breathing that is required according to the demand. Secondly, they breathe out too hard on the exhalation and breathe inadequately on the inhalation thereby creating an imbalance. This subsequently results in not fully and properly regulating the breath with the movement, both on the inhalation and the exhalation. I also notice their posture isn't as upright as the typical athlete's. One or all of these factors might occur, but I notice these differences clearly and obviously between the fit athletes and the unfit person.

Athletes can perform continuously and tirelessly because of their physical training. I am aware that there are numerous factors that constitute this training, but obviously I will focus only on the breathing component. I spent many years questioning all different kinds of athletes around the world. Some of them have been world champions in their chosen sport. We discussed at great lengths how they specifically breathed while performing, and, where possible, they demonstrated. At the same time, I had many unfit people wanting to learn how to improve and control their breathing so they could ease the frustration and struggle they experienced during exercise.

As an experiment, I decided to teach unfit people to breathe the way an experienced athlete breathed during performance. Firstly, I emphasized that they maintain upright posture the whole time they exercised. Apart from all the positive benefits proper posture gives, it also allowed them to breathe more freely, as they could move their diaphragm and ribs without any restrictions. Next, I made them aware of the importance of making sure they deepen their breath and showed them how to regulate their breathing for their particular chosen activity.

I was astounded by the results achieved, and so were my clients. People who had previously struggled with exercise were able to increase their duration of training without stopping or feeling exhausted. (How much they improved varied depending on the individual.) Interestingly, as time went on, they self-improved their overall performance. They could detect and feel if their posture, technique and breathing were correct or incorrect.

Obviously, muscles and other important factors need to be developed if you are to become fitter, and this takes time. But I don't believe anyone would argue the importance of breathing appropriately for exercise as a component to overall performance. Just ask any athlete. And also ask them this: if they were to breathe in a shallow manner, or even halve the amount they typically breathe for their sport, could they perform as well? Athletes tell me that there is a specific breathing pattern and volume that is in accordance with their movements, which helps them perform properly and move with ease.

Relaxing into the movement and practicing an ideal way of breathing while you are exercising gives you an opportunity to at least stop the unnecessary struggle and execute your motions much more easily. This gives you the opportunity to improve the quality of your performance and the duration if you so desire. As a result, you will gradually upgrade your fitness levels. To summarize, here are a few important factors that will help you to exercise most efficiently:

1. Proper posture with an emphasis on keeping upright the whole time
2. Correct application of technique for each sport/movement
3. Breathing deeply and appropriately according to the demand

If you put into play the lessons you have learned in this book, you will soon approach exercise like a fit person—that is, you will draw in the required amount of breath and fully regulate your breathing. Once you have established the basic principles and practice them a bit, you will soon find a corresponding lift in every aspect of your performance.

So if you are unfit and usually give up trying to exercise because you always feel you battle with it, be assured that you can exercise without strain or pain. If you put some effort into applying the three factors mentioned previously, I guarantee that you will approach physical activity with more enthusiasm. Like so many others, you will also realize that exercise makes you feel more alive and it can be enjoyable! You did it naturally in your childhood, and you loved to move back then. Imagine recapturing that feeling and rediscovering your body's instinctive need and desire to be active.

Unfortunately, unfit people mistakenly think that they are uncoordinated, or too old, or simply do not have the ability to exercise and never will. They are wrong! I have worked with 60-year-olds who have managed to improve their breathing and fitness in a short space of time. So believe me, everyone who is basically healthy has the capacity to at least participate in minimal exercise without struggling—even if it is swimming or brisk walking. Once you learn how to breathe correctly as you move, you will be able to exercise with ease, and if needed, you will easily and naturally increase your duration. And don't be surprised if you find you are actually enjoying yourself in the process and feel like you could do more!

In his book, *The Oxygen Breakthrough,* Dr. Sheldon Hendler from New York City explores the impact of breathing as well as exercise and food on the functioning of the body's cells. In addition, he writes about how, in his experience as a medical practitioner, he found that some of his patients were having trouble exercising because of improper breathing, poor quality eating and other factors. He believed that their exercise programs were causing them more harm than good.

After following his advice, these same people found themselves so energized that they were able to exercise comfortably and without the struggle they had previously experienced. Some of them even went on to compete in marathons. Dr. Hendler believes that, for the average person, moderate exercise is best for health. But of course you can be more active if you approach exercise wisely and safely. His main point is exercise, but for optimum results, exercise correctly by breathing properly. He also believes maintaining a healthy diet plays a crucial role in achieving results.

Dr. Hendler states:

We have become a nation of shallow, thoracic-chest-breathers, neglecting the primary muscle of respiration: the diaphragm. Most of us do not use the diaphragm the way it was intended to be used.

And

Mastering proper "outer" breathing is one of the most important things anyone involved in aerobics can achieve. Optimal outer breathing enhances endurance by reducing the amount of oxygen you need to consume at any given workload.

When you are exercising or performing any demanding physical activity, you will find it helpful to:

- use (deep) throat breathing for both the inhalation and the exhalation.
- emphasize the diaphragm as your focal point to breathe in and out of. Draw in large amounts of good quality breaths mainly to the diaphragm (also the chest if desired, but not chest only).
- maintain correct form at all times (even if you feel tired).
- keep the whole chest and rib cage area up and open as much as possible.
- allow the rib cage to freely move inward and outward as much as possible.

Unless instructed by a qualified trainer, you should not:

- hold on to your breath.
- breathe directly in and out of the upper chest in a shallow manner.
- breathe out so hard that the inhalation is obviously weaker and shorter than the exhalation.
- let your shoulders, sternum and upper chest move up and down unnecessarily, or drop downward.
- allow your posture—in particular your shoulders and upper chest—to slump at any time.

Regulating the breath technique

Case study using swimming

I recall joining the local pool for swimming lessons. I was still in the early stages of exploring breathing in relation to movement and exercise and was eager to try out a few concepts I had learned from athletes. Within a short time, I was able to swim non-stop for well over an hour. I would finish feeling invigorated and I felt I could have continued swimming. My coach was baffled! In the end, given the short time I had been coached on technique, he said the breathing was a significant factor. The other ladies who were learning to swim with me complained they could swim only a couple of laps before they felt exhausted. They assumed it was because they were unfit and aged 50-plus. They asked me to show them how to swim so they wouldn't struggle during exercise and feel so breathless.

First, I made sure the ladies were moving properly and executing the basic swimming techniques correctly. Next I showed them how to regulate their breathing for each movement. Within a week, there was a noticeable improvement. The average improvement ranged from two "struggling" laps to 10 "energetic" laps. But the best part of it all was that they felt refreshed and invigorated throughout the session as well as afterward. Needless to say, from that point on, they began to look forward to their swimming sessions.

APPLYING THE TECHNIQUE

Swimming is used here as an example of regulating the breath, but the basic principles can be applied to other similar sports. The first aspect you need to look at is the length of the stroke. If you refer to the illustrations, you can see that one stroke refers to the movement of one arm as it moves through the water. For the purpose of learning, you must go slowly, so I will use a count of 10. You can speed the pace up later if you want to, but only after you have grasped doing it properly and slowly. Let's look at each stage by breaking down each movement.

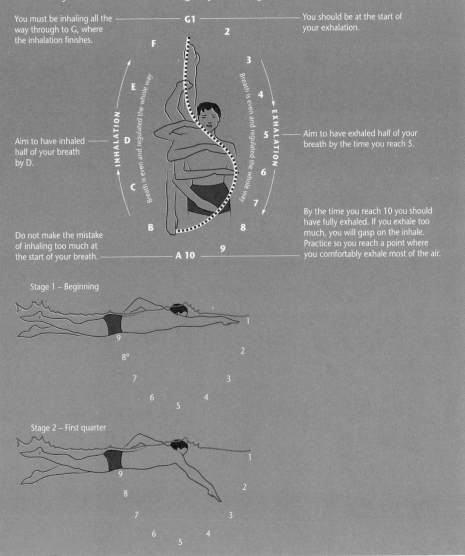

You must be inhaling all the way through to G, where the inhalation finishes.

You should be at the start of your exhalation.

Aim to have inhaled half of your breath by D.

Aim to have exhaled half of your breath by the time you reach 5.

Do not make the mistake of inhaling too much at the start of your breath.

By the time you reach 10 you should have fully exhaled. If you exhale too much, you will gasp on the inhale. Practice so you reach a point where you comfortably exhale most of the air.

Stage 1 – Beginning

Stage 2 – First quarter

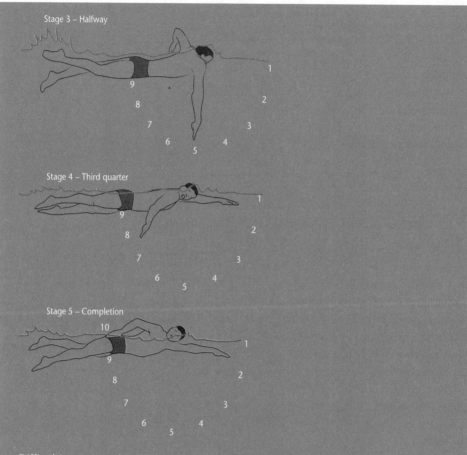

Stage 3 – Halfway

Stage 4 – Third quarter

Stage 5 – Completion

Difficulties occur when either the inhalation or the exhalation, or both, have been applied inappropriately. Regulating the breath throughout the whole phase of the inhalation and the exhalation is the most significant concept to understand. If you gasped for your inhalation at the beginning, or at any other stage of your inhalation, one or all of the following happened:

• Your exhalation was too weak.
• You did not exhale fully.
• You exhaled too quickly and/or abruptly.
• You exhaled with unnecessary force.
• You breathed out too much, too soon.
• You held your breath at the beginning, during or at the completion of the movement.
• You made an improper changeover from inhalation to exhalation and/or exhalation to inhalation.

Try the following before you attempt swimming in the water:

1. **Breath only**—Inhale and exhale the exact amount of breath that you estimate is required for the movement.

2. **Movement**—Stand up and go through the arm motions exactly as they should be done. Concentrate only on the precision of the movement and do not be concerned with how you are breathing (although make sure you do not hold it at any point).

3. **Breath and movement**—Now join both breath and swimming movement together. If you do not breathe in fully and properly, it will affect the way you exhale; consequently the whole act of swimming will become a strain and a struggle. As previously discussed, it is not necessarily because of your lack of fitness, technique or your age but because you are insufficiently supplying your body with the right kind and amount of breathing required. If you breathe adequately and appropriately, at least you can execute the technique much more efficiently than if you are struggling to breathe. It is so important to match your breathing with your movements.

I have had so much positive feedback on application of this technique when applied to different sports. There has been an endless amount of people (including the unfit and the elderly) reporting to me that they instantly improved, not only with their technique, but also their stamina. In regards to swimming, there seems to be an instant improvement with many people doubling the laps they were previously doing, and with much greater ease.

Particularly for swimming, practice the concept of regulation until you master it. The main problem to be aware of is the common mistake of inhaling and exhaling too much too soon. The ideal is to pace out the breath and movement making sure neither are abrupt or erratic. Once you have mastered the basics, then you can try these:

1. **Speed up your pace**—If you want to speed up your pace, then reduce your count. For example, complete your inhalation and its corresponding movement by the count of four or five, and move faster.

2. **Increase the number of your strokes per breath**—apply the same procedure, but complete the exhalation and the count by the end of the increased number of strokes. So, if it was two, the first of the two strokes would consume half of the total exhalation, and the second stroke the other half of the breath. If there are three strokes, the breath is divided into three, so that by the time the third stroke has finished, the exhalation has been fully completed. This requires a bit of working out, so I suggest you practice it for a little while out of the water first.

Can you see the importance of inhaling and exhaling properly and fully? By making sure you regulate and fully exhale, a vacuum is created. This will automatically result in the body drawing in a big, deep breath from A to G (refer to the diagram on page 131). The mistake is to gasp and breathe in only for as long as A and B, which is a very common habit with inexperienced swimmers. You have an opportunity to draw in a large amount of air by applying two components:

1. Use a good quality and deep throat breath for both the inhalation and exhalation.
2. Inhale over the whole stroke, i.e., from A to G, and exhale over the whole stroke, i.e., 1 to 10.

Make sure you do not "passively" pull in the breath. If you do not put enough gas in your car, what happens? When you exercise, you demand a lot from your body so how can a limited passive breath give you enough energy to execute the movement? Here is your opportunity to give yourself a huge boost of energy! Really energize yourself by opening your mouth wide and intentionally drawing in a deep breath for the whole inhalation phase.

By now you understand that a good quality and appropriate exhalation is required for exercise to continue properly and efficiently. By also making sure the breath is deep and regulated, you have a few essential and significant components that will give you the opportunity to begin improving your whole manner of exercising.

Balancing breath technique

This technique is helpful if you become breathless easily whenever you exercise. The basic principle of the technique can be used for any sport but is particularly useful for aerobic activities such as walking, jogging, swimming, biking and aerobics.

What I commonly observe with unfit people when they are exerting themselves is that they tend to breathe one dose of inhalation and usually triple the amount they exhale. Is it any wonder they become breathless and tire so quickly? How can the body have the energy to continue a demanding task if the breath is not balanced in a healthy manner? What inevitably happens is the imbalance becomes greater until there is barely enough breath to sustain the demand of the movement. The only choices are to continue to struggle or stop the activity altogether.

But how do fit people breathe when performing an activity? They immediately draw in a substantial amount of breath, and at the same time, simultaneously fall into an appropriate rhythm. Unfit people take too long to sufficiently deepen their breath, consequently not drawing in enough to meet the demand. Also, the breath is typically erratic, therefore interfering with the ideal rhythm. They can actually deplete stored energy by their insufficient breathing and feel worse if they continue to exercise. And some medical experts advise that breathing inappropriately can impose some constraints on the heart. So it does not make sense to struggle with exercise, risk your health and on top of that, end up feeling exhausted. On the other hand, by breathing ideally for the activity and using proper form, you can enjoy exercising, enhance your health and energize your body so that you end up feeling invigorated—like a healthy fit person does.

So the fit person continuously and appropriately breathes deeply and easily from the beginning of an exercise session and throughout. The lungs and rib cage naturally open up, and there is more room for even more breath. I have witnessed thousands of people—even those who are unfit and loathe exercise—learn how to appropriately breathe for sports and exercise. And unless you have a health problem, there is no reason why you can't learn.

Applying the technique

A step

You can apply the "balancing breath" technique to other activities, but we will use walking as an example. As I will be referring to "steps," first, let's define what I mean by "a step." Picture yourself walking and imagine your right leg is behind you and your left leg is forward. A step is the point from the right leg being behind and moving forward until it is placed in front with the left leg now behind. This is considered "a step." The left leg coming forward and landing in front is considered another step. *Your step/s MUST be synchronized with your breathing* otherwise the technique will not work.

Changeover

This is the smooth transition between inhalations and exhalations. I will also refer to this term regularly. Actually, not only is it part of the technique, it is also a very important component of basic breathing. I spoke about four parts that constitute breathing. Apart from inhalation and exhalation, there are the two stages in between, which I referred to as "transitions." I will now give you a brief exercise to help you understand the difference they make and their necessity while you are exercising endurance. (Once again, these four stages happen fully and automatically with fit people, whereas, unfit people don't always allow them to happen fully.)

Inhale and exhale three times without pausing in between the inhalation or the exhalation. Now try this: see if you can *gradually* and *smoothly* blend your inhalation over to your exhalation. It should not feel or sound abrupt at any point. Your aim is to make sure the changeover is so gradual that it would be difficult to detect at what point the inhalation stops and the exhalation begins, and where the exhalation finishes and the inhalation begins. Repeat this a few times until you can feel the whole four stages are happening fully and smoothly without your gasping or being abrupt at any point. I will be explaining this whole procedure in greater detail.

However, if you can do the above exercise properly at this stage, it will make the whole technique significantly easier as you are exercising.

Let's begin

First try to imagine yourself performing this technique, then try it physically. Picture yourself slowly walking along step by step. Instead of breathing in too much and too quickly and then breathing out too hard and allowing your shoulders and upper chest to drop downward, try the following exercise.

STAGE 1—INHALATION

Begin with an upright posture and maintain this throughout the whole exercise period. Proper posture is crucial and the technique will not be as effective unless you remain upright the whole time.

With the mouth relaxed and open, use a deep, good quality throat breath, and pull the breath down into your diaphragm area. It is extremely important that you inhale as deeply as possible and draw in ample amounts of air over four steps.

The quality and strength of the breath needs to be regulated and consistent from the first step right through to the fourth. Each breath should be the same in sound, depth and rate. The common mistake is to pull in too much breath on the first step, which will leave you with weak breaths for the remaining steps that you are doing while inhaling.

You need to make sure the breath is reasonably strong, but do not make it so strong that it lasts for only one or two steps. As you keep practicing, you will be able to breathe in a good quality, voluminous breath for at least four steps.

STAGE 2—FIRST CHANGEOVER

Your next task is to change over to the exhalation. This is the main changeover. A common fault is to breathe out too abruptly after inhaling. When the inhalation is completed, you need to consciously create a smooth transition over to the beginning of the exhalation. You must not hold your breath, but allow for whatever time is needed to *gradually blend* the inhalation and exhalation together.

STAGE 3—EXHALATION

There is a common automatic tendency to push out far too hard on the exhalation when an activity or any kind of demand is placed on the body. But in order to keep on exercising properly, you must regulate the flow of the exhalation and the inhalation. If you do not control your breath and body, they will control you, and you will struggle to keep exercising or be forced to stop. If you want to continue exercising for a lengthened period of time, *do not allow the breath to be exhaled in a forceful manner,* even if this is how you have always breathed during exercise.

It helps if you keep reminding yourself that it is the proper balance of inhalation and exhalation and oxygen and carbon dioxide that gives you the required energy to perform easily. Keep a watchful eye on how much breath is actually being drawn in, compared with how much is being expelled, and *continuously aim to keep the breath appropriately balanced.* Draw in enough air to sustain the demand of the movement, and keep the exhalation regulated and under control. This is one of the most important components, and it is crucial to master if you wish to exercise properly.

STAGE 4—SECOND CHANGEOVER

There is a brief period after the exhalation when there is another transition period, but this time it is from the completion of the exhalation over to the beginning of the inhalation. It is only for a step or two, so you need to be prepared to start pulling in the inhalation quite early for this stage. You will find that the changeover is a lot shorter and not as comfortable as the changeover after the inhalation. This is natural because of the tendency for your lungs to recoil inward following inhalation. As you have already experienced, it is your body's survival instinct to inhale when the exhalation is complete, and even more so when *fully* expelled. Even though exhalation is normally a passive process, remember that your body has the capability to actively control it if you choose to, especially during physical exertion.

It is up to you to control and regulate the exhalation so that you do not breathe out so much and so hard that you are forced to gasp for your inhalation.

While the breath should be expelled adequately from the lungs, do not make the mistake of exhaling to the extreme. You need to avoid gasping because an abrupt inhalation inevitably results in a short or shallow breath. Work both the inhalation and the exhalation together as a unit, along with the changeover stages in between. We all marvel at how endurance athletes can keep performing tirelessly and yet still manage to consistently control their breathing. Athletes also continuously keep their posture upright, so until this process becomes a habit, constantly remind yourself to do the same—really open your chest and make sure your diaphragm is free, allowing it to perform its duty to breathe fully and powerfully during exercise.

The four stages are the basic formula. As you practice, you will be able to efficiently regulate the required amount of air flowing in and out at any given time, in any activity.

The main points to emphasize are:

- Pull in voluminous amounts of deep, good quality throat breaths.
- Regulate the exhalation.
- Stop the constant shallow breathing into and out from the upper chest.
- Do not drop your shoulders or upper chest when you exhale.

If you resolve these points, and practice the four-stage procedure until it becomes habitual, you should find you can control your breathing much more efficiently whenever you exercise.

The energizing breath

The energizing breath is a way of breathing that can help increase stamina while you are exercising. It can give you a feeling of being energized as you are training, rather than making you feel depleted of energy.

First, it is important for you to learn how to master the ability to adjust the volume of your breath from as soft as possible to make it as dynamic as possible (see page 55). Every all-around athlete has mastered this with great expertise. *In developing this skill, you will be able to appropriately adjust how you breathe in a variety of activities.*

The "energizing breath" is an excellent technique to use when you feel like you are starting to lose control of your breath and/or are becoming exhausted. It can be used, firstly, before you approach a strenuous activity; secondly, during the strenuous activity, and thirdly, afterward, during the recovery period.

1. Let's say, for example, that you are about to walk, jog or cycle up a hill. Unfit people find themselves breathless very early on the incline. Because you are going to use a lot of energy in order to reach the top of the hill, the technique can be applied before approaching it. This will help to compensate for some of the energy that will be used for such a demanding and strenuous activity.

2. Using the technique as you make your way up the hill isn't easy when you are inexperienced at either the breathing technique or climbing hills, particularly if you are unfit. However, after you practice a few times, you will notice a difference in your ability to gradually increase the distance and yet still feel reasonably good. This indicates that you are applying the technique properly. (If you are puffing and feeling too breathless at any stage, it is better to stop and revive yourself before going on. As you become fitter, you will improve and eventually you won't have to stop at all.)

3. When you reach the top of the hill, you may be struggling to regain your breath, depending on your fitness level, how steep the hill is, and how hard you pushed yourself. Spend the first few minutes deliberately recovering your breath so that

you are not panting furiously. Using a good quality throat breath, inhale as deep as possible. Aim to draw it into the diaphragm and lower rib cage area, and if you need to, the upper chest as well. But make sure you do not only breathe in and out of your upper chest, as it will take you a lot longer to recover and you may not recover as efficiently as when you fully use the diaphragm and breathe in a deeper manner.

APPLYING THE TECHNIQUE

The teeth must either touch gently or be only slightly apart. This creates a sieve and prevents the breath from rushing in all at once, allowing you to control and regulate your breathing. Make sure you use a good quality throat breath to pull the breath in as deep as possible. Then slowly but surely, release the exhalation with control. The duration of the exhalation will vary, but the main thing to watch is that you do not allow yourself to breathe to the extreme end of your exhalation. Just breathe out to the point where you feel you have fully exhaled.

It is crucial that you keep the chest and shoulders upright, especially when exhaling. The tendency is to drop them. Even when the activity you are doing is strenuous and very demanding, persist in reminding yourself to never drop your upper chest area while exercising and recovering, no matter how tired you are. It would be better for you to stop exercising and regain your breath before continuing, or breathe more deeply. You will need to slowly build up your fitness level and your ability to use the technique while you are exercising and during the recovery period afterward.

As you become more experienced, you will automatically work out what intensity of breath is needed at different times. (You can always go back to the exercise on page 55 to help you with this.) Experiment and work out what is right for you. It does take practice—but when you find that unbearable tight sensation in the chest is no longer being felt (or is at least significantly reduced), you will agree that it's worth it.

Specialized breathing training for fit athletes

A fit person naturally breathes at a high standard when exercising. Fit people:

- understand and perform all the essential factors for exercising efficiently.
- automatically breathe deeply and adequately for the activity they are performing.
- breathe appropriately as soon as they begin exercising and for the duration of the exercise.
- regulate their breathing with their movement fully and properly.
- utilize the full strength of the diaphragm, which consequently strengthens it even further.

Athletes can compliment their cardio-respiratory fitness training with advanced and specialized breathing training. The emphasis is to predominately work the diaphragm muscle to breathe deeply, along with the abdomen and upper chest, as opposed to mainly working the upper chest. As this method of breathing does not exhaust the body, it can be practiced while resting and/or in a recovery phase. And it is especially helpful for injured athletes who can do the techniques when they cannot practice their normal training.

Breathing training can help athletes to relax and calm themselves before or during important events. Every competitive athlete knows that for optimum performance, a certain amount of mental and physical relaxation is essential prior to competition. I have received quite a bit of feedback that relaxation breathing has been extremely helpful for calming of the nerves before competing.

Athletes are also taught how to *consciously* control and strengthen their diaphragm, allowing them to breathe even deeper into their lungs and minimize any unnecessary upper chest movement. This results in their being able to regain their breath quicker and more efficiently, thereby decreasing their recovery time. Some changes were subtle, others significant, but change did occur. Their newly acquired ability to relax deeply consequently increased their flexibility. This is usually the biggest notable improvement and a great relief for all athletes, but in particular, for those who feel muscle-bound and extremely inflexible.

I enjoy working with athletes because they are so dedicated to improving themselves. These days, they are looking for every edge possible to give them an advantage in the tough competitive world of sports. According to what they have told me, it became obvious that specific breathing training can give athletes an opportunity to work their diaphragm and breathing from a different angle. Some athletes find certain exercises that are part of the specialized program (i.e., designed specifically for them) quite difficult. Some exercises are so challenging that they can't be executed properly until certain muscles have been trained in a specific way.

I am often asked who do I think is the best breather? For the males, my answer is Robert Harvey, who has won the prestigious Brownlow Medal for AFL football twice in a row. Why? Because he is the most *instinctive* breather I have ever come across. He instinctively changed his breathing to suit every exercise including the ones for flexibility—a true athlete in every sense of the word. In the female category, Danny Roche, who won gold in women's hockey at the Olympics in Atlanta (1996). She was able to work the breathing techniques superbly, mastering all of them with great ease. She is truly an inspirational athlete in every way.

Basic tips for athletes

There are six main areas you can work on:

- Learn to consciously control your whole manner of breathing by using the diaphragm proficiently and practicing good quality throat breathing. The mega breath (inhalation and exhalation) and the power breath are particularly good for athletes.

- Make sure you can actually hear your breathing, constantly checking that the sound is of a high quality. For example, when you are practicing relaxation breathing, it should sound smooth, not inconsistent. When you are power breathing, make sure the sound isn't weak, but rather is strong and gutsy!

- Experiment as much as possible on varying the intensity, volume and rate of your breathing. Especially master the ability to soften your breathing, which helps you relax and increase your flexibility and allows you to stretch your body comfortably.

- Learn to move your rib cage inward and outward powerfully without obvious movement from the shoulders and upper chest, and with minimal movement from the abdomen. (Note: This is a breathing exercise. You will probably breathe differently when exercising.)

- Practice breathing exercises when you are still, in order to develop your diaphragm and breathing. Make sure you are relaxed and either sitting or lying down.

- Do the flexibility exercises at least once a day. This is especially important for muscle-bound athletes who constantly feel tightness in their chest, back, abdomen and rib cage area.

Stress management and relaxation

There are many books and tapes available about stress management and relaxation, and it is not my intention to cover the subject in great detail here. But as breathing has an important role in stress management, we will take a brief look at it.

Stress is generally seen as a negative trait in this day and age. However, it is a necessary part of our lives and it's an instrumental component of achievement on most levels. It's only when we try to suppress stress or simply don't deal with it adequately that the damage is done.

Paradoxically, the more relaxed you become, the more energy and vibrancy you will experience. Continually carrying tension is tiring and depletes our energy supplies. But when we allow ourselves to relax and let go of the tension, those supplies are refueled and we feel energized.

Our natural state is relaxed. Take a look at a child, for example; notice how free babies and children are in their bodies. If we are full of tension and uptight, then we have interfered with our natural state. And we need to introduce some measure of relaxation into our lives to return us to our natural state.

Practicing relaxation is important so that anxiety breathing, as a result of stress, does not become habitual. The only way relaxation of the mind and body works is to release the stored tension that we have. Relaxation is not something you can try hard to achieve. Simply "letting go" is a more effective approach, and is ultimately the only way the body can relax.

Bear in mind that it can take a while to master total relaxation. Guided tapes can be beneficial. Again, I want to point out that this chapter does not provide a detailed set of instructions on how to relax; I simply want to introduce some basic tips for improving your relaxation process. Before we get started, let's take another look at the relaxation breathing pattern. (See page 41.)

For maximum benefit in a minimum amount of time, try the combination of long, slow, smooth throat breaths with calming and relaxing thoughts. This should relax your whole body and mind very quickly.

Abdominal/diaphragmatic breathing patterns are connected to the relaxation response of the mind and body; whereas upper chest breathing is connected to the stress response. If you observe your (or others') breathing during a stressful situation, you will notice that either you are shallow breathing into the upper chest or you are struggling to hold on to it. Either way, it will feel very erratic and seem as if it is "stuck" in your chest area, which is quite the opposite of the free flow of breath when you are in a relaxed state.

A very important component is the sound of the breath. A smooth, harmonious throat breath is mentally calming. If you allow the sound of gentle breathing to relax you mentally, you will very efficiently fall into a physically relaxed state. Simply focus on making the breath as smooth, long and gentle as possible. To achieve a very deep relaxation, follow the soothing sound of a rhythmical breath.

To achieve a deep state of relaxation, a quiet atmosphere is needed. I realize that this is not always possible, but try to find a quiet environment when you are in the initial learning stages of your relaxation sessions. As you become more experienced, you will learn to relax even in a noisy environment or stressful situation.

I was forced to test my own ability to relax a few years ago when I was temporarily living in the U.S. My sister has two pit bull terriers, and one day while everyone was out they turned on me. I instantly focused on my breathing to keep me calm and relaxed. I did not know what to do, but in order not to upset the dogs further, I decided that I had to stay calm and show no fear. This was not easy, as one of the dogs, which had already bitten me on the leg, moved in and began barking viciously, right near my ear. At that moment, I thought I was going to be ripped to shreds by the pair of them.

I somehow managed to get near the phone and called emergency services. But I figured that by the time anyone got to me, it would be too late as it appeared I would be mauled. I talked to the woman at emergency services for some time. All the time I was breathing slowly and gently. I was trying to keep my voice low and calm, despite the fact that the operator herself was panicking because by now both of the dogs were moving in on me and barking ferociously at my ear!

After 45 minutes of this living nightmare, I began to tremble a bit. Then the same dog that had bitten me before, bit me again—this time on the arm. Thankfully, it ended at that point as I picked up a chair to defend myself, which unexpectedly scared the dogs, who sprinted from the room (lucky the door was open!). So I miraculously escaped unharmed, apart from the nips.

Later, I was told that perhaps I would not have been so lucky if I had not appeared calm and relaxed throughout the experience. If I had showed the dogs fear, I don't even want to think about what could have happened!

This experience taught me that it is possible to relax (or to at least appear relaxed) in the most stressful of circumstances. I believe that it was my previous relaxation training that taught me to draw on that deep well of calm inside that I know exists. Also, the sound of the throat breathing was pacifying for my nerves. It was physically and mentally calming and something my mind could focus on to enable me to keep relaxing, no matter how nervous or frightened I felt.

THE RELAXATION BREATH

The key to relaxation is lengthening and softening the breath and totally letting go on the exhalation. Follow these steps:

1 As you listen to your relaxation tape or as you move through your own relaxation routine, always begin by taking deep breaths. Deepen each breath as much as you can by breathing slowly with each inhalation and especially when exhaling.

2 Pull the breath in gently for as long as you comfortably can and pause. Aim to lengthen your exhalation and take time to fully expel the breath to the very end without forcing it.

3 Allow yourself to go limp with each exhalation. With each breath, go deeper and deeper into relaxation. Gradually, your bodily tension will melt away.

A fundamental and most important key for relaxation is to pace your breath so that it is long and slow. If your method of becoming relaxed does not include a slowing down and deepening of the breath, you will not be able to fully and properly relax. It has been proven with biofeedback machines that you can only reach a deep state of relaxation when the breath is rhythmical, harmonious, smooth, deep and gentle.

Tips

- If you are trying to relax by using words alone, not only will it take you longer, but you might not attain a very deep level of relaxation. The mind and body need deep, rhythmical breathing to fully relax.
- There should not be any abrupt movement or tightening of the breathing muscles. Even your face, neck, back and shoulders need to be consciously relaxed.
- Make sure you are throat breathing rather than sniff breathing.

So how can you use relaxation breathing in stressful situations? You should:
- acknowledge that you are stressed and become aware of how you are breathing.
- mentally tell yourself to calm down and think of calming thoughts.
- try as much as you can to control your breath and slow it down.
- soften and lengthen each breath as much as possible.

It is important to keep the breath moving in and out and imagine it is moving through your whole body, rather than allowing it to stay stuck in the chest area. Obviously this is not easy when you are angry or frightened, but it can help reduce that uncontrollable, destructive anger or distress that can cause tension to build up. The main aim is to at least try to change how you would normally react.

Coming from a Greek culture, I know all too well about fiery emotions! For some of us, rage, temper and verbal expression are a part of who we are. You may always be that way by nature, but I do believe you can learn to control anger most of the time rather than let it control you! I don't believe anyone can claim that they never feel stressed, hurt or angry. We are all human and sometimes our emotions do get the better of us. When this happens, it is helpful to try to use a relaxing breathing technique and calming thoughts. In fact, it can be implemented in any facet of your life. Professional business people have told me that they have found it helpful for calming their nerves during stressful meetings and students find it helpful for exams.

I often use it while waiting in heavy traffic and bank lines or any time I need to feel calm and relaxed. If you feel an argument or a dispute is about to erupt, try using the common advice of breathing deeply and counting to 10. You will feel much more grounded and hopefully may be able to avoid many confrontations.

EXERCISE TO OVERCOME STRESS

If you find you become stressed too often, I suggest you try this exercise. Pinpoint the particular times in your life that make you feel stressed, angry, uptight, agitated, nervous, impatient and so forth. Now imagine yourself in any one of those situations. See yourself mentally calming down and at the same time taking long, deep, even breaths. (If you are in public, you can breathe in such a way that no one will notice.)

You might find it difficult to do at first but persist. It becomes easier with practice and will eventually become an automatic response. You will find yourself choosing the healthier and more harmonious way of dealing with various stresses of life.

Coping with pain

As I mentioned in the introduction to this book, I first learned how to cope with physical pain during my teenage years of training in the martial arts. I realized that if, as a female, I wanted to cope in this male-dominated field, physically and mentally, I had to find a way to cope with intense pain. I was surrounded by men who had mastered the handling of extreme pain and I was awed by their ability to do this.

My karate instructor taught me how to breathe properly when striking and I always trained a lot more effectively when I used this powerful method of breathing. As time went on, I realized that if I exhaled really hard at the peak of pain, somehow the pain was reduced. I did not understand why at the time, but I knew that if I was struck and happened to be inhaling, it was much more painful. Needless to say, it did not take me long to make sure I exhaled hard any time I was struck.

The diaphragm can be strengthened when it is specifically trained, and I had quite a few instructors whose training methods involved power breathing and also included methods that strengthened the diaphragm. After a lot of practice, I mastered the ability to breathe so powerfully that I could detach myself from pain by precisely synchronizing a really strong exhalation at the exact moment of a strike. I became an observer of pain and eventually reached a point where I was not so afraid of it.

Because of this fear of pain, most women tend to gasp and hold on to their breath when they are experiencing it. Holding your breath makes you more receptive and sensitive to pain; therefore, it feels more intense. When I taught women how to give and receive a strike in martial arts training, they all found they could strike harder without hurting themselves when exhaling dynamically. They also found it was less painful to receive a strike when they exhaled powerfully. So a solution is to exhale as hard as possible at the exact moment the pain occurs. But what if the pain is a continuous one, such as a cramp, headache or a labor contraction?

I have been told that various techniques work for different types of pain, so it is a matter of finding what suits you. For example, basic deep breathing has helped with headaches. The belly breath (see page 115) is ideal for prolonged pain—keep exhaling continuously in short, sharp bursts for as long as the pain continues. The relaxation breath (see page 144) may be useful if the pain is so intense you find it difficult to relax. The aim is to at least subdue the pain. Apart from using a breathing technique, do whatever you feel you need to do in order to help take your mind off the pain, for example, perhaps you could lie or sit in a specific position or use a hot water bottle.

I must issue a health warning at this point: any recurrent pain must be referred to a medical physician. Pain is a warning that something in your body has gone wrong and requires urgent medical attention.

EXERCISE

Think of a pain you personally experience that you would like to reduce, for example during sports or when you are having an injection. Assess the kind of pain it is—sudden or prolonged—then try to figure out how to breathe so that you can find the most relief. For example, your exhalation should be at its hardest at the exact point that the needle is inserted. Practice breathing so that when the real pain hits, you are ready for it and know what kind of breathing to do.

I have talked to a number of women who have used various breathing techniques during labor, who all claim it helped make the contractions bearable. I have also found these techniques good for people who avoid exercise because "it hurts." When the people breathed in a specific way, they found the exercise quite bearable and were astonished to find that they actually even enjoyed it.

If you try using the breathing techniques and they don't work, don't give up. It could be that you haven't quite grasped how to exhale hard enough, and/or you did not synchronize the breath with the pain. Or you may need a different technique for your particular pain.

Breathing during labor

Women often find that each birth experience is different. Depending on a number of factors, the duration and intensity of each contraction, and the time between them, can vary. So neither aspect can be predicted, and you need to allow for variation. The only certainty is that there will be a contraction and a period of time before the next one. These will change as the stages of labor change.

As you will be unsure of when the next contraction will happen or what it will be like, it helps if you familiarize yourself with the whole process. Try to gain a general idea of contractions and how you might handle them physically and mentally in respect to duration and intensity. Consider their varying range of times, for example, compare a contraction that lasts for 40 seconds with one that lasts 1.5 minutes. Also think about the intensity of a contraction, and be mentally prepared for the various changes in intensity throughout labor.

Common positive feedback suggests that you take advantage of the time between contractions by regaining your breath, while mentally and physically relaxing as best as you possibly can. It helps if you keep preparing for the next contraction while you are doing this.

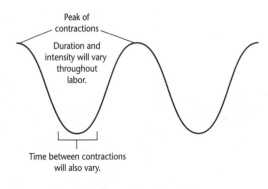

Peak of
contractions

Duration and
intensity will vary
throughout
labor.

Time between contractions
will also vary.

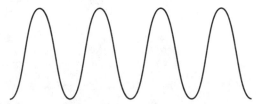

Toward the end of labor, contractions will be at their most intense,
and the time between will be shorter. There is a buildup, which
you need to be both physically and mentally ready for.

There are many reasons whey childbirth can be painful. I was given the honor
of assisting a friend of mine, Angela, through her labor. Because of that experience
helping Angela to breathe properly, I came to understand one of the reasons why
childbirth can be painful for most women—and yet others find the whole event
quite tolerable. It is natural that many women experience excruciating pain, and I
write this section in the hope that breathing training can ease that pain for some.
(I haven't experienced childbirth myself, so the information is provided by women
who have.)

As the contractions are so exhausting, the period between can be used for
reviving yourself using the relaxation breath (see page 144). This will help you to
replenish your breath and allow you to mentally center yourself, in readiness for the
next contraction. The following three points can make all the difference between
having a painful labor or a bearable one, and I suggest you practice them before
going into labor:

1. Coping with physical pain (see previous chapter).

2. Regulating breath with movement (see page 130).

3. The belly breath (see page 115).

In the opinion of the ladies I have worked with, all the techniques in the world will
not help you as much as learning how to throat breathe with precision and strength.

Mentally, this technique will keep you calm and centered, give you energy and help you to cope with what seems like never-ending pain. Throat breathing gives you the opportunity to breathe really deeply, using the full strength of your diaphragm. This means you can control your breathing so that you will be able to work "with" the contractions rather than resist them or feel overwhelmed by the intensity of them. I have emphasized the importance of the exhalation, but you also need to be aware of the inhalation. During labor, women are encouraged to breathe abdominally. Once again, use throat breathing to inhale slowly and deeply, particularly between contractions to help calm and center you. The absolute worst thing you can do is inappropriately hold on to your breath, unless instructed to do so. If you remember one thing, remember this: B-R-E-A-T-H-E throughout your labor.

The support person

It helps if the person you choose to be with you during your labor learns as much as you do about breathing. This is because during the contractions, the pain can be so great that it is highly likely that you will forget to breathe, and you will also forget all of the techniques that you have practiced!

That's when your support person can remember for you. They need to:

- continually remind you to B-R-E-A-T-H-E.
- calm and relax you whenever you need them to.
- motivate you to get through those seemingly endless contractions.

Thankfully these days most men want to be involved in the birth process and are excellent supporters. The women I have worked with told me that it made a huge difference having their partners there, breathing with them every step of the way. I would like to share some of their experiences with you here, in the hope that they may help you.

Angela and me

We spent about six months prior to the birth practicing and experimenting with different techniques. In order to prepare for the contractions, Angela practiced and perfected the belly breath. The duration of the average contraction varies, depending on a number of factors, but Angela practiced so she could do this technique properly for just over two minutes. Over the months, I really fine-tuned her breathing style. By the time she was due, we both felt confident that she would be able to breathe well throughout labor.

When Angela's contractions started in the hospital, I encouraged her to throat breathe, firmly and gently. I encouraged her to relax and suggested that she breathe as deeply as she could. I also gently breathed near her so she could hear the noise, which would remind her to keep breathing.

As the intensity of the contractions progressed, I kept my eye on her breathing to make sure that it was synchronized perfectly with the intensity of each contraction. This is where it is crucial that the support person is in tune, otherwise their (breathing) support will be of no benefit. If the woman loses control of the breath, then she reduces her ability to control the pain. And so I made sure that Angela's exhalations were at their strongest when the contractions were at their peak.

I will always remember the look on Angela's face when the baby gracefully emerged. She looked at me and the first comment she made was that she had been able able to overcome the intense pain. When I spoke with her afterward, we spoke in great detail about the experience and what she had found particularly helpful. Angela told me that in order to keep the pain under control, she needed to be constantly aware. It was the breathing more than anything else that she felt kept her in control. We both agreed that the throat breathing in particular gave her emotional and physical strength.

In Angela's own words:

The breath provided the link between my inner and outer self, and you need both because you have to stay conscious to release the pain of the contractions. The breathing also helped me to concentrate and stay focused the whole time and gave me inner and outer strength despite the overbearing pain. Hearing Sophie breathe continually, along with her verbal reminders, made all the difference for me. It helps to be as well prepared as possible, by practicing the breathing and feeling confident with it. It is crucial that your support person constantly reminds you to breathe, and it does help if they can be close to you, loud enough for you to hear.

When Angela asked me to be her support person, I found it helpful to study the contractions so that I would understand the rhythms, peak, timing and intensity of pain. This experience was without doubt one of the best of my life, and I am sure the world stood still at the moment when the baby's head came out facing me. I thank Angela from the bottom of my heart for sharing such an unforgettable and awesome event with me.

Emma and Annie

Emma is a friend of Angela's, and she happened to be pregnant at the same time as Angela. Emma chose another friend, Annie, to be her support person. They all ended up doing a breathing course together with me, so we were all in baby mode. Emma said that when she was doing a lot of deep breathing, she could feel the baby moving and kicking. We laughed as we assumed it was all the oxygen the baby was receiving that made it wake up and feel full of life. Annie had an excellent grasp of the breathing techniques, and it ended up being an absolutely wonderful experience for both of them. Emma stated that after all the deep breathing during her labor, she actually ended up feeling wonderful. So much for painful births.

Linda and Glen

Linda and Glen were expecting their first baby. Glen wanted to help Linda through it all, and they came together to do a breathing session with me. I only managed to spend one session with them, yet even that seemed to be enough for them to grasp the importance of specific breathing techniques to help them through labor. When they came to see me with their brand new baby, born on New Year's Day, they told me how much the breathing techniques had helped them. Linda also said that having Glen remind her to breathe continually was a tremendous help.

Loanna and Tony

For the delivery of her first baby, Loanna's experience was so painful that she blacked out and missed out on the actual birth. Her one wish was that she would stay conscious for the birth of her second baby. Loanna diligently practiced all the breathing techniques that I taught her and felt prepared mentally and physically. Tony also trained with her. Loanna was ecstatic with the outcome of the second delivery. Not only did she stay totally conscious throughout, but she said it was a much easier experience and practically painless compared with the first.

Loanna told me that even though she knew how to breathe correctly, having Tony there to remind her to keep breathing was very important and a great relief during the contractions. They brought the baby to class and gave us a firsthand report on the whole experience. Tony actually demonstrated how he placed himself right over her face and in a loud tone, encouragingly said, "Breathe Loanna, b-r-e-a-t-h-e." The world needs more support people like Tony!

Sue

Sue had to have forceps used for the birth of her first baby. She told me that for the delivery of her second, it was her (new) obstetrician who helped her with her breathing. She said she could not believe the difference it made to the labor.

I realize that the first time is usually the worst and thereafter labor is naturally easier because all the relevant muscles have been previously stretched. But I have had women tell me that every labor was excruciatingly painful for them. With the help of proper breathing, you can at least ease the pain so that each experience is a bearable one.

Specific health conditions

Insomnia

Imagine waking up refreshed, rested and feeling like you have had a good night's sleep. This is one of the wonderful positive side effects of breathing deeply. A number of people have told me that after practicing lots of good quality deep breathing, their quality of sleep improved. Others told me they slept soundly and adequately for the first time in years.

Unfortunately, not everyone experiences a good night's sleep every night, as any insomniac will tell you. A night for them consists of restless and endless tossing and turning and results in even more frustration when they have very little sleep. When training insomniacs during a private breathing session, I have found that they tend to have a common breathing problem. When consciously working with the breath, the connection between mind and body seems to become confused. When insomniacs are following my instructions for the first basic breathing technique, most of them abruptly change either the breath or body movement or sometimes both after a short time.

Most insomniacs find the (breathing) instructions difficult to follow precisely, even when I am slowly demonstrating each step. Initially, they follow the instructions correctly and then at some point, the messages become mixed—usually without the person being aware that they have changed incorrectly.

The good news is that eventually all of them managed to follow the instructions correctly. Some found an immediate improvement in their sleeping patterns; others took a lot longer. A few found no improvement at all in their sleeping pattern so there are no guarantees that breathing training will help insomnia. But all the people I worked with felt that the effects of relaxation generally helped them feel better. They also used different breathing techniques in other areas of their life, such as when exercising.

The most helpful advice I can give to insomniacs is to understand methods that assist them to breathe deeply and rhythmically, so they can carry that into their sleep. Learning how to breathe in a way that is in harmony with sleeping soundly plays a fundamental part in improving the quality of sleep. Even if you wake up during the night, then at least you can spend the time practicing deep breathing exercises rather than being stressed out about not sleeping.

Whether or not you are an insomniac, it is to everyone's advantage to learn the best way of breathing for a restful sleep. If you constantly breathe in a shallow and erratic manner, it could take a while for your body to wind down after a day of stressful breathing. So it would be helpful if you begin to breathe in a relaxed manner a little while before retiring. Then, by the time your head hits the pillow, you will eventually fall into a deep and restful sleep. When you wake up, you will feel rejuvenated and refreshed.

Asthma and other respiratory problems

Asthma is a huge problem in our society today, even in young children. The problem is not just that an asthmatic has to inhale a copious amount of drugs in order to breathe properly, but also that they feel like they are going to suffocate and/or die when an attack hits them. The positive news is that even asthmatics have the ability to learn how to breathe deeply just like anyone else. In fact, I was surprised myself that in many instances, they were able to improve more than some people with a normal and healthy respiratory system. So if you are an asthmatic, you will be happy to know that, regardless of how many years you have had asthma, you can improve and learn how to breathe fully and correctly.

At this point, I must emphasize that the breathing training is not a substitute for your asthma treatment. Your doctor must keep advising you. The fact is that you may always need to use your inhaler.

I believe learning to breathe consciously is important to asthmatics for two reasons:

1. To lay the foundation for a healthy attitude toward breathing. (You will feel more at ease and comfortable with your whole manner of breathing.)
2. In the event that you are caught without your inhaler, to help you breathe sufficiently and stay as calm as possible until you reach your medication.

When asthmatics do not have their inhalers during an attack, they immediately panic and begin to tell themselves they cannot breathe without the inhaler. Some believe they will die (and unfortunately some do). This, understandably, causes a great deal of stress and will result in an even more constricted and panicked manner of breathing.

If, on the other hand, you can assure yourself that you are able to control your breathing at least until you get to an inhaler, then you have a better chance of not making the problem worse.

By taking some deep abdominal/diaphragmatic breaths through the mouth and controlling your exhalation by breathing out slowly and gently, you can assure yourself that you will be fine (you can use the relaxation breath explained on page 144). The gentle and calm breathing will put you at ease until you can be helped. Panicking is literally the worst thing for you to do, as it will make your breathing worse by becoming more constricted. If you have never had any breathing training and have not learned how to control your breathing, I can understand why you would panic. But if you have had instructions on how to control your breathing, in an emergency such as an attack, you will, at the very least, have more confidence to endure the ordeal until all is well again.

It would be beneficial if you could make it a priority to do some form of breathing training regularly to help keep your breathing healthy and your diaphragm extra strong. If your doctor approves, you might like to choose one of the suggested programs. Singing also seems to help some asthmatics. And while swimming helps for reasons other than breathing, a number of people have told me they had asthma as children, took up swimming and never had a problem again. Breathing training may or may not help you through your worst moments, but at least you can use it, like everyone else, for exercise and relaxation.

Smoking

Almost every smoker at some point in time complains about how hard it is to give up smoking. They are baffled because they often have strong willpower in other areas of their lives, but when it comes to smoking they just can't quit. This makes them feel weak, frustrated and hopeless. No matter how determined they are, they repeatedly fail to give up smoking. Everyone has one or more bad habits that are hard to give up (myself included), so we all share this frustration. This section is not intended to make you feel bad about being a smoker, but rather look at how you could possibly smoke less, or even better . . . give it up permanently!

First of all, it is well documented that nicotine is a very addictive substance. Some people have told me that, for them, smoking is harder to give up than some drugs! Giving yourself a hard time about not being able to quit will only add to your stress. A more positive way of approaching the problem is to seek help from the experts.

Smokers often ask me if breathing training could help them give up smoking. I do not think any one thing will necessarily work for everyone, and the successful people are those that ask for help when they are ready to quit. A lot of support and different programs are offered these days to help people give up smoking once they have made the commitment to stop.

I have found that after learning how to breathe fully, some smokers were able to give up smoking permanently and without any desire to begin again. It does not work for everyone, but it is worth at least giving it a try as a supplement to other methods.

The first person I tried my experiment on was my sister. After 10 years of smoking, she gave up permanently, and the best news is she also lost the desire for it. That was more than 10 years ago.

DEEP BREATHING

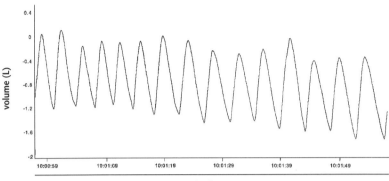

1 minute

ERRATIC BREATHING

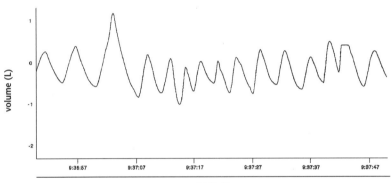

1 minute

The above diagrams illustrate long, slow, deep and even breathing, which relaxes you, and erratic breathing, which stresses you. While carefully observing how people breathe when they smoke, I noticed there was not one person who did not change the way they breathed when they smoked, including puffers. One reason why smoking helps people to relax is because they change from erratic breathing to longer, deeper and smoother breathing in order to draw the smoke in and expel it. Taking a long, slow, deep and even breath is very calming and relaxing with or without a cigarette. So it would be natural that if you tried to give up smoking, you would probably feel agitated or stressed because you had stopped the relaxed breathing you have become accustomed to. Is it any wonder that you would feel a strong desire to smoke again, especially if the addictive nicotine is also still in your system?

So if you really are ready to give up smoking, you could try the following method, which has been used with success. First, you need to be aware that it takes a while for the nicotine to leave your system, so the craving that you have in the initial stages will be more intense. This craving will subside as time goes on. Secondly, especially for the first few days, try to keep your awareness on your breathing as much as you can. Constantly breathe in a rhythmical, smooth and relaxed manner, similar to when you are actually smoking.

When the urge to smoke hits you, take deep, calming breaths and remind yourself that the craving is only temporary, and it will be easier to resist the temptation as time passes. A day will come when you just won't even desire a cigarette. When the urge hits you again, immediately think of all the negative consequences. Just imagine how disgusting your lungs will be—black and suffocated—if you continue to smoke. Stay committed to your goal to make your breathing and lungs as healthy as possible. Tell yourself you can do it. Keep thinking about the thousands of others who have done it, so why not you? They are no different from you. They are not any stronger willed or better than you. If they can do it, so can you. They had the very same urges you have and yet overcame them. If you make the commitment and set a goal, you will find the inner strength to give up permanently. Those who have succeeded in overcoming any bad habit say that positive self-talk and the continual reinforcement of their goals is crucial for success. You know what the negative effects of smoking are, but also visualize the positive effects not smoking will have on you. Picture yourself with healthy pink lungs, glowing skin and all that extra energy! Just think about how much better you will feel by not touching a cigarette.

The ideal aim with any addiction is to not desire the action or substance. I am a strong believer in changing the association in your mind so that you form a positive picture in your mind of what you do want (healthy lungs and easier to breathe) every time the urge to smoke hits you. If you use only willpower and try to force yourself to stop, either you will become very stressed and start to smoke again or you will transfer the addiction to something else.

As I mentioned, the first person I worked with on giving up smoking was my sister, Marie. We started a program of detoxification to rid her body of the built-up nicotine. At the same time, when the urge to smoke hit her, I asked Marie to take long, slow, deep and even breaths until the urge subsided, which was usually about three to five minutes later. This method reprogrammed her mind so that instead of reaching for a cigarette to relax her, she would take full deep breaths. Finally, the association of smoking for pleasure had been permanently changed so that she couldn't stand the smell of smoke! It was like a miracle.

After that experience with Marie, I have met so many others who were heavy smokers for decades and gave up permanently. These people have inspired others who desired to give up smoking. My hope for every smoker is to permanently lose the craving to ever want or need to smoke again. Whatever effort it takes to give up smoking is worth it. Like thousands of others, you can make the decision to quit, join a program and help overcome your urges by B-R-E-A-T-H-I-N-G your way through them—and have a smoke-free healthier life!

Epilogue

We have reached the end of the book, but for many of you "relearning" how to breathe is just the beginning. This book has been about breath—the awesome miracle that gives us life. While we can survive without food and water for a period of time, all forms of life depend upon a constant supply of air for breath in order to stay alive. Breath is universal. The spark of life was given to all of us at birth through our breath, so it is worth thinking about my original question: How many of us have consciously utilized our breath to its maximum potential?

What I have offered to you in this book is information to help you not only become an all-around breather, but to also improve your posture and flexibility, allow you to relax effectively and exercise with more joy and ease. The act of breathing is involved in everything we do. As your awareness and breathing skills increase, you may discover better ways of breathing or at least feel an improvement in all activities in your life.

You may need some time to acquire the new skills required to change old habits. Allow this change to occur gradually. If you are only used to walking, then you wouldn't go running for an hour, so take the same precautions with your whole approach to breathing training. I have witnessed some dramatic improvements after a few simple changes, but for long-term benefits you must be patient and practice.

Once you have learned to become an effective breather, you will begin to experience new sensations and feel a difference in your breath, body and actions. You will know when your breathing has improved, not only because you breathe much more deeply, but also because the sound is like a gentle breeze rather than an abrupt sniff of air. Once you can consciously strengthen and relax the appropriate muscles, you will begin to feel your breath effortlessly flow gently and powerfully without strain or struggle—this is the breakthrough from shallow to deep breathing.

Allow for variations in your breathing patterns. The nature of breathing is that it is subtle and often changeable. It reflects all our emotions: we breathe a sigh of relief, belly laugh when we are happy, breathe shallowly into our upper chest when we are stressed. The most important information you need to be clear about is that shallow upper chest breathing is associated with stress and that deep rhythmical abdominal/diaphragmatic breathing is associated with relaxation of the mind and body. Keep in mind that rhythm, depth and quality of breath are very important.

Remember that conscious breathing can be practiced anywhere and at any time—obviously the ideal environment is out in the fresh air. If you live in a highly polluted area, use the breathing techniques during exercise, and practice deep breathing exercises indoors—it is crucial for city people as they desperately need to utilize their full lung capacity to compensate for the pollution and lack of natural movement in their lives. Regardless of where you live, breathing training is still necessary for everyone because it teaches you to control your breath for all your activities.

I continue to be fascinated by breathing and still explore it because it enhances all aspects of my life. Breath is timeless. The incredible sensation I felt when I took my first really deep breath 20 years ago is the same sensation when I take a deep breath today, and I'm sure this will be the same sensation for another 20 years.

A wonderful lady I have known all my life, Joan, had this to say after becoming aware of the importance of breathing training: "You can see how much learning how to breathe correctly influences a happy and healthy life, so do yourself a favor and breathe for a good long life!"

Oprah Winfrey once suggested on one of her shows to choose five things that you are grateful for, and if you can't think of five, you can always choose breathing.

We can choose to utilize the breath effectively in a myriad of ways or to not consciously use it at all. By learning how to use the breath to its maximum potential, you can stop depending on insufficient shallow breaths to get you through life. Increase your lung power; it is only a breath away.

My final wish to you is to be inspired to fully B-R-E-A-T-H-E FOR LIFE.

Index

Cooling breath, 115
Costal (thoracic) breathing, 27–28
Coughing, 20
Counting, 119

D

Deep breathing, 3, 5, 6, 9, 31, 35–40, 41,
    54, 71, 72, 111, 146, 151, 152, 155, 158
  positive benefits of, 5, 6
  types of, 35–38
Diaphragm, 27, 37
  exercise, 92–93
  training, 92
Diaphragmatic breathing, 30, 31, 35, 37,
    38, 39–40, 61, 88–110, 142, 154, 159
  overview of, 95
  versus abdominal breathing, 38–39
  See also Abdominal breathing.
Diaphragmatic exhalation, 96–101
Diaphragmatic inhalation, 101–106
Double pause exercise, 59

E

Energizing breath, 138
Erratic breathing, 41, 155
Exercise, lack of, 9–10
Exhalation. *See* Expiration.
Expiration, 30
External breathing, 2, 31, 32, 111, 121–122

F

Flexibility, stretches for greater, 75
Food, effect of, on breathing, 11
Forward-bend stretch, 80–81
Four stage breathing, 112

G

Genetics, effect of, on breathing, 10

H

Harvey, Robert, 140
Hendler, Sheldon, 129
Hendricks, Gay, 12
Horizontal stretch, 76–77

I

Ibuki breathing, 52
Ideal breather, being a, 23
Illness, effect of, on breathing, 11
Imagery exercise, 76
Imagination, using, 61
Inhalation. *See* Inspiration.
Injury, effect of, on breathing, 11
Insomnia, 152–153
Inspiration, 30
Intercostal muscles, 27
Internal breathing, 120
Isolation exercise, 92

L

Labor, breathing during, 147–151
Le Boyer, Frederick, 7

M

Martial arts, 121
Massage, 82–84
  abdominal, 83
  neck and shoulders, 82
  respiratory muscles, 83–84
  ribs and diaphragm, 83
  self-, 82
Measuring posture, 67
Meditation, 120
Mega breath, 108–109
Mega exhalation exercise, 110
Mega inhalation exercise, 109–110
Mouth breathing, 22, 32
Muscular tension, effect of, on
  breathing, 9

N

Natural breathing, 16–18, 22, 23, 24, 48
  healthy, 18
  testing at rest, 17–18
Neck and shoulders massage, 82
Nose breathing, 22, 32

O

Oxygen Breakthrough, The (Hendler), 129

P

Pace, 55
Pain
  coping with, 146–151
  effect of, on breathing, 11
Pelvic tilt, 94
Pollution, effect of, on breathing, 10
Poor quality breath, 3
Posture, 64–70
  poor, effect of, on breathing, 8
Power breath, 56, 116–117
Power breathing, 37–38, 115

R

Reading exercises, 119
Reflex controls, 19–20
Regulating exercises, 60–61
Regulating the breath, 114
Relaxation, 120
Relaxation breath, 55, 144–145
Relaxation breathing, 35
Respiration, 27
Respiratory distress, signs of, 18
Respiratory muscles massage, 83–84
Respiratory problems, 153–154
Respiratory system, 27
Rib cage, rigid, effect of, 9
Ribs and diaphragm massage, 83
Roche, Danny, 140

S

Scale breathing, 113
Scuba diving, 121
Self-massage, 82
Self-regulating responses, 19–20
Shallow breathing, 4, 33
  indications of, 17
  See also Upper chest breathing.
Side-bend stretch, 78–79
Sighing, 20
Singing, 120
Single pause exercise, 59
Smoke, effect of, on breathing, 10

Smoking, 154–156
Sneezing, 20
Sniff breathing, 32
  exercise, 52
Sound exercises, 118
Stick stretch, 79–80
Stress
  effect of, on breathing, 8
  exercise to overcome, 145
  management, 142–143
Stressful breathing, 34
Stretching, 71–81

T

T'ai chi, 39, 121
Tension check, 75
Throat breathing, 32–33, 52–57, 58, 76, 116, 130, 134, 139, 143, 149, 150
  exercise, 53–54
Thoracic. See Costal breathing.

U

Ujaii breathing, 52
Unhealthy breathing habits, reasons for, 1–2, 7–11
Upper chest breathing, 30
  shallow, 33–34

V

Vertical stretch, 77–78
Volume, 55

W

Whistling, 119
Wind instruments, 121

Y

Yawning, 19
Yoga, 120
Yoga breathing, 35–36

Z

Zones, 29